EXIT WOUNDS

A Survival Guide to Pain Management for
Returning Veterans and Their Families

Derek McGinnis

U.S. Navy Veteran, Iraq War

with Stephen R. Braun

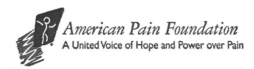

American Pain Foundation
A United Voice of Hope and Power over Pain

WATERFORD
LIFE SCIENCES

Published by Waterford Life Sciences, Washington, DC
Cover and book design by Arisman Design Studio

For information about how to partner with APF
on distribution of this book, contact:

Tamara Sloan Anderson, MSW
Director of Strategic Development
AMERICAN PAIN FOUNDATION
P: 413.628.4510
Email: tamara@painfoundation.org

For information about ordering books
and discount pricing on bulk orders, go to:
www.exitwoundsforveterans.org/bookorders

The development of *Exit Wounds* and its companion
website were made possible by the generous support of
the following organizations and companies:

- Disabled American Veterans (DAV) Charitable
  Service Trust
- Elan Pharmaceuticals
- Purdue Pharma L.P.
- Wyeth Pharmaceuticals

Contents

Preface: Scott M. Fishman, MD, President and Chair, American Pain Foundation   **1**

Introduction: Winning Your War on Pain   **5**

1. To Hell and Back: Derek's Story   **15**

2. Coming Home in Pain   **41**

3. The Anatomy of Pain   **59**

4. The Consequences of Untreated Chronic Pain   **71**

5. Your Mission: Improve Function   **89**

6. Your Arsenal of Treatment Options   **99**

7. Exercise: A Key to Pain Relief   **131**

8. Treating the Emotional Wounds of War   **147**

9. Getting the Help You Deserve   **169**

Epilogue: A Call to Action   **185**

Resources for Veterans in Pain and Their Families   **188**

Endnotes   **193**

Acknowledgments   **196**

About the American Pain Foundation   **199**

Preface

One of the ironies of the recent wars in Iraq and Afghanistan is that improvements in body armor and battlefield medicine have enabled many more soldiers to survive traumas that would have previously been fatal, but more are coming home with serious, complex, and persistently painful injuries. The physical injuries are often accompanied by the invisible wounds of battle, including: anxiety, depression, and posttraumatic stress disorder (PTSD). Overcoming the physical wounds as well as the emotional scars of battle is necessary to heal the whole person, relieve the experience of pain, improve function, and maximize quality of life for both the individual and the family.

Chronic pain, whether suffered by individuals in the civilian or military community, is a special kind of hell. It erodes quality of life, self-esteem, even the will to recover and resume a full life. Chronic pain can persist well beyond the time when physical injuries have healed, with serious long-term effects on the individuals, their loved ones, caretakers, and extended families.

The American Pain Foundation (APF) developed *Exit*

1

Wounds, and its companion website, in response to the unique needs of our military personnel returning home in pain, as well as for their families and caregivers. Veterans who answered the call to service and who have endured grievous harm to body and soul *deserve the best pain medicine available.* The goal of *Exit Wounds* is to arm veterans and their families with the information and resources they need to advocate for the quality of pain treatment they deserve.

Despite all the advances in battlefield medicine, pain management has lagged behind other specialties. For instance, veterans who have endured amputation will find a remarkable array of high-tech prosthetics available. Yet the treatment of phantom limb pain, which afflicts more than half of veterans with lost limbs, is evolving more slowly. *Exit Wounds* is designed to educate readers about the most effective pain care options now available, and to help veterans and their families to navigate a complex and often overworked and underfunded healthcare system.

Exit Wounds offers practical guidance, authoritative medical information, and hope. The author, Derek McGinnis, is a voice for all veterans struggling to reclaim and rebuild their lives. His story, movingly narrated in the first part of this book, shows how a severely wounded veteran with the support of his family recovered a rich and rewarding life in the wake of a near-death, life-changing injury and painful rehabilitation. Derek was supported in this effort by APF's expert medical staff, specialists in pain medicine for veterans. And the book's companion website, www.exitwoundsforveterans.org, provides military personnel, veterans, and their families with a constantly updated online resource.

For APF—an organization that raises public awareness, provides education, promotes research, and advocates for improved access to effective pain management—answering the unmet needs of our active military and veterans in pain is more than a priority. It's an imperative. Over the past two years, we have worked tirelessly on Capitol Hill to advance legislation to ensure treatment for our active military and veterans in pain. These include the Military Pain Care Act of 2008, which was recently incorporated into the 2009 National Defense Authorization Act, and the Veterans Pain Care Act of 2008, which became part of the Veterans Healthcare Policy Enhancement Act of 2008. APF's military/veterans outreach programs are extensive, including online support networks to combat the isolation of chronic pain, such as the Freedom from Pain Campaign and PainAid for Military/Veterans.

Exit Wounds signals APF's expanded partnership with and support for all of our military and veterans who suffer persistent pain. I commend Derek on sharing his story of hope and inspiration. This is a timely and invaluable book, one that all active military members, veterans, family members, caregivers, and many within the civilian community will benefit from reading. I also commend each and every one of our active military and veterans for their selfless service to our country, and the brave resolve of those facing the challenges of recovery from injury and pain.

Exit Wounds is a small measure of our admiration and gratitude.

Scott M. Fishman, MD
President and Chair
American Pain Foundation

Introduction:
Winning Your War on Pain

*When you come to the end of your rope, tie a
knot and hang on.*
—FRANKLIN D. ROOSEVELT

For wounded veterans, overcoming pain is the final battle: hand-to-hand combat with an adversary we were never trained to fight. Pain can be an elusive, stubborn, and
sadistic enemy. If you or a loved one has battled chronic
pain, you already know this firsthand. I do, too.

I was wounded while serving as a Navy Corpsman
with the Marines 3rd Light Armored Reconnaissance
Battalion in Iraq. During the second battle of Fallujah in
November 2004, my Humvee ambulance was hit with an
IED that nearly killed me and wounded several others in
the vehicle. I was saved by the tremendous skills of many
military doctors, nurses, and others—many of whom I
never actually met. But my recovery was hell—as you'll
read in the next chapter. I experienced pain beyond anything I had previously endured. There were times when I
gave up, gave in, sat down. But those were temporary set-

backs. I kept fighting, and eventually got treatment that worked. Today I can walk, run, ride my bike, take care of my boys—live the life I choose. I'm not totally pain-free—nobody is—and not everything's perfect. I have my struggles, like any other married man with two kids, a job, and a full schedule of courses. But they are normal struggles and, for that, I am blessed.

I've written this book because when I was struggling with pain, there was no guide, no map, no mentor to steer me through the minefield I was navigating. I relied on the love and support of my wife and family and my own determination to master the military healthcare system, deal with all of the nonphysical aspects of chronic pain, and figure out how to get the care and treatments that I needed.

But this book isn't just for injured veterans. Pain—especially unrelenting chronic pain—affects everyone around the person feeling the pain, and recovery is almost always a group journey—a family journey. That's why this book is as much for spouses and children, parents and partners, and extended family members and friends, as it is for the service members themselves. The wounded need to recover, and so do those around them. Like my father, David McGinnis, says, "As Derek healed, we healed."

Because my family was so crucial to my survival and recovery, I've recruited them to help tell this story and to help guide others through the sometimes terrifying obstacle course of pain. At the end of each chapter you'll find a section called "The Family Journey" where I'll make suggestions for how family members and friends can support wounded veterans. You'll also be hearing from my wife, Andrea, and my parents, Barbara and David, who share lessons they learned from their experiences of helping me fight pain and regain my life.

I've also drawn on the voices of other veterans—from past wars as well as the ones we're fighting today—to help express the many challenges that wounded warriors face when they come home in pain. You'll hear these "Voices of Survival" throughout the book, and you may recognize yourself or a loved one in these profiles in courage.

As part of my personal journey back from pain, I decided to train and to run in triathlons. As any triathlete will tell you, the most important part of the race isn't below the waist, but between your ears. Your mental attitude more than your body gets you across the finish line. And you can't finish if you give up. That's probably the central message of the book, and it's what I tell other veterans nearly every day: Don't give up. Don't give up hope that your pain will eventually fade and that you can recover a life worth living, and be redeemed. Don't give up on yourself or the people who matter most to you.

Fighting pain demands the same level of patience and stamina as doing a triathlon. You can't sprint through the whole thing, and you can't sprint through recovery and rehab from severe combat injuries. You have to pace yourself. You may hit walls of pain. You may have moments of despair—as I did. But if you keep going, keep pushing, you're going to win the war against your pain. That's when you'll know you've made it home, alive and whole, no matter what you may have left behind on the battlefield.

How This Book Can Save Your Life

Think of this book—and the companion website (www.exitwoundsforveterans.org)—as a survival guide. Use it however it serves you best—for inspiration, for information, for hands-on advice about how to navigate the healthcare systems available to you (DoD, VA, and civilian).

Whether you're a veteran in pain or somebody who loves one, your mission going forward is to learn as much as you can about pain, treatment options, the harmful consequence of leaving pain untreated, and the steps you can take to get the best care possible. Most of all, you need to become an advocate for the pain treatment you deserve. You need to learn how to be assertive without antagonizing your support team, and how to fight smart instead of just flailing away with brute force. The fact is, the care is out there; you just have to know where to look for it and how to go after it.

People with untreated or poorly treated chronic pain often cannot live the lives they want. Their pain and their constant search for relief undermine their relationships with those they love, their ability to work effectively, and, inevitably, their self-esteem. Chronic pain often leads to sleep disorders, emotional distress, anxiety, and depression. Unaddressed, these problems can lead to a dangerous spiral of despair; some may even consider suicide. Tragically, in 2008, 128 service members killed themselves—the highest suicide rate since the military began keeping statistics in 1980. Chronic pain is not the sole cause of suicide, of course, but it can be a critical factor in the tailspin that can precede it.

It doesn't have to be this way. Throughout this book I will emphasize the importance of getting help for pain *as rapidly as possible*. Research shows that unrelieved pain, regardless of its initial cause, can become a disease unto itself, damaging the nervous system and causing abnormal changes in pain pathways of the nerves, the spinal cord, and the brain. We now know that it doesn't take long for pain to become "hardwired" in the body. When it does, the consequences are serious, both for the person in pain and those around him or her.

In the civilian world, complaints about pain are the number-one reason people go to the doctor: pain afflicts more Americans than diabetes, heart disease, and cancer combined. The same facts apply—but carry an even greater sense of urgency—to the men and women returning from military operations in Iraq and Afghanistan. A recent study of soldiers enrolled in VA Polytrauma Centers showed that:

- ✪ More than 90 percent have chronic pain.
- ✪ Most have pain in more than one part of the body.
- ✪ Pain is the most common symptom in returning members of the military.

Complicating the care and treatment of wounded veterans is the fact that pain is often poorly understood by many healthcare professionals. Unfortunately, the science of modern pain management is still relatively young. That means many physicians practicing today received little, if any, training in pain management during medical school and have not kept abreast of all the exciting developments that have taken place in the field over the past decade.

It should go without saying that by putting themselves in harm's way for their country veterans have earned the right to the best possible treatments, the highest standards of care, and the most comprehensive of services. And, certainly, the military healthcare system has taken great strides in recent years to achieve these goals. Unfortunately, it's not there yet—as portions of my own story will illustrate. Still, the system is far more advanced than is often portrayed in the media; and every day the knowledge of effective, innovative pain management practices spreads a little further among clinicians working in these massive and complex federal health institutions. That's encouraging news, yes, but it doesn't mean you may not have to fight for your right to pain treatment, or the right kind of pain treatment.

That's the primary purpose of this book, to help you achieve your personal pain management goals. I'm convinced that, armed with the information and tools provided in this book, you can reduce your pain and restore function in the vital areas of your life: work, love, recreation. Without resorting to medical jargon or citing needless technical details, I'll tell you what I've learned about the different types of pain and the many treatment options that now exist to deal with it. You'll come to realize that beating pain is about much more than pills, IVs, or surgery. Pain is complicated. People are complicated. The strategies you use to combat pain must, therefore, be able to help you unravel these complications. Your strategy must be flexible, tailored to your specific needs, and broad enough to cover both mind and body.

More than laying out the facts about pain and pain medicine, I also hope this book instills in you a healthy attitude toward pain management. You will hear me say this repeatedly: *You* are the critical key to success. Your doctors cannot simply wave a magical medical wand and "fix" you. Rather, you must take command: View your doctors as the expert consultants you "hire," who offer their skills and recommendations and who will work with you at every step on your journey to overcome pain. The responsibility for success rests, ultimately, on your shoulders.

Your military training can help in this mission. Call upon the courage, discipline, and drive instilled in you by your training. Whether you need to advocate for yourself or a loved one, or fight for the attention and treatment you deserve, always follow the command structure, be respectful, and do your homework. This was the approach I adopted, and I've seen it work for others.

Remember: the race is not always to the swift, but to those who keep on running.

EXPERT ADVICE

To ensure the accuracy of the medical information in this book, I enlisted help from two expert practitioners of pain medicine: Brenda Murdough, MSN, RN–C, and Rollin M. Gallagher MD, MPH. I also drew from the wealth of pain information and educational resources offered by the leading nonprofit organization working for people in pain: the American Pain Foundation (APF). The medical information in this book reflects their combined wisdom and experience.

Brenda Murdough, MSN, RN-C is a clinical nurse who, for the past decade, has specialized in pain management for the Dartmouth–Hitchcock health system in Keene, New Hampshire. Her understanding of the challenges veterans and their families face when they come home from war also comes from personal experience: her son served 15 months in Iraq, her brother served in Operation Desert Storm, her husband is a retired Army colonel, and her niece recently returned from Afghanistan.

Rollin M. Gallagher MD, MPH is the former director of Pain Medicine at the Philadelphia VA Medical Center, professor in pain medicine at the University of Pennsylvania, and deputy national program director for Pain Management for the Veterans Health System. He has been a tireless advocate for and pioneering practitioner of expert pain treatment for veterans. His efforts include serving as principal investigator of a VA study with the U.S. Department of Defense examining the long-term impact of early, aggressive treatment of pain in troops severely injured on the battlefield. Dr. Gallagher became interested in the phenomenon of pain early in his career when he was working as a family doctor, delivering babies in the Colorado mountains. After a nurse from Paris introduced him to the Lamaze breathing techniques, he witnessed women able to deliver babies without medication and with greater control over their labor outcomes. The experience planted a seed. Later, he studied why some patients do not recover from chronic pain, and he began to appreciate the complex nature of chronic pain: that it has mental, social, and neurological components, which, combined, make it a formidable public health challenge.

The American Pain Foundation (APF), founded in 1997 by leaders in the pain community, has established itself as the leading patient advocacy organization for people affected by pain, as well as those who care for them. APF's mission is to improve the quality of life of people living with pain, by raising public awareness, providing practical information, promoting research, and advocating to remove barriers, and thus increase access, to effective pain management.

As the largest pain organization serving consumer needs, APF several years ago launched the Military/ Veterans Pain Initiative to reach out to the growing number of veterans, members of the military, and their families. This initiative:

✪ Provides free educational materials and peer-to-peer support.
✪ Reduces feelings of isolation.
✪ Ensures that the unique needs of returning and retired service members are adequately addressed.
✪ Empowers those living with pain to seek appropriate pain care for themselves and their comrades.

APF also steadfastly advocates on behalf of veterans for comprehensive, multi-disciplinary pain treatments. Encouragingly, in the fall of 2008, two major pieces of legislation were signed into law that will help do just that. These bills call for improving pain care and increasing pain research in both the Department of Defense (DoD) and the Veterans Administration (VA). The VA is required to provide: (1) necessary pain management for long-term chronic pain disabilities, and (2) education and training to VA healthcare professionals on how to assess and treat pain.

APF has also created the website companion to

this book, www.exitwoundsforveterans.org, which contains more detailed information about most of the topics covered in *Exit Wounds*. The site offers extensive resources and authoritative, up-to-date information about types of pain and specific pain treatments, as well as links to other valuable websites and communities. The APF website also features an online support community and discussion boards called PainAid. There are sections within PainAid that are specifically dedicated to veterans and their family members. Thousands of people log on to this site to talk about the issues they face and to share solutions that work.

1. To Hell and Back: Derek's Story

American flags mean a lot to me. I fly one from my house in the small town of Waterford, California. On one wall of my home office are three glass-faced triangular frames, each holding a folded American flag used in the military funerals of my two grandfathers and a step-grandfather. On another wall of the office is a flag covered with hand-written notes from 19 of my fellow Marines. The American flag represents the values of freedom and service that I believe in, that I went to war for, and that I sacrificed for.

But three years ago, I was losing my battle with chronic pain. The scene I'm about to share testifies to the power of pain to grind down a human soul.

Picture this: It's a chilly March evening in Bethesda, Maryland. I'm in a wheelchair, rolling myself along a path on the sprawling grounds of the National Naval Medical Center, where I was being treated for my injuries. It was dusk, and a Navy sailor was lowering the flag from a pole—a ceremony called "evening colors." Ordinarily, like any service member, I would stop, face the flag, remain

silent, and salute until the "carry on" signal was given. That
was the tradition I learned and, until that evening, rigor-
ously upheld. But at that point, I didn't care. I was coming
back from a meeting with my medical team—and nobody
was listening to me. I was in such pain, and nothing they
were doing was working. I was totally pissed off, muttering
to myself, "Fuck it, fuck this place, I'm outta here." I rolled
right through "colors" and went inside. It was something
I would never do normally, because you think of all those
people who have gone before you, and how they fought
for that flag. That's what "colors" is all about, thinking
about the people who have gone before you. That evening
though, I was too consumed with my own battle to stop.

This chapter is the story of how chronic pain drove
me to the point where I no longer cared about one of the
most sacred things in my life. It's also the story of how,
with the help of dozens of professionals and the deep love
of my wife and family, I finally beat the pain, rebuilt my
life, and began helping others who are struggling with the
same issues.

★★★

I grew up in Fremont, California, a suburb of Oakland
on the eastern side of San Francisco Bay. As a kid I was
athletic. I loved surfing, skimboarding, and skateboarding.
In school I played defensive end and tight end on the foot-
ball team, and defense on the soccer team. Track was my
favorite sport, because it was individual—you're compet-
ing with yourself, trying to beat yourself.

Whenever I got interested in something, I locked on to
it and worked hard. I liked biology, for example, and got
A's. But, honestly, aside from sports, my friends, and my

high school sweetheart, I didn't focus on much in school. By my junior year, I was itchy. I didn't know what I wanted to do with my life. I knew I wasn't ready for college, but I wanted to leave the house, be independent, do my own thing.

With veterans on both sides of my family, I figured the military was a good bet. I wanted to be a Marine, but my mom, Barbara, was pushing hard for me to learn a skill that I could build on when I came out. I had always been interested in emergency medicine. Problem was, the Marines have never had their own medical corps, like the other branches of the military. As an advance attack force that had evolved out of the Navy, the Marines have historically relied on Navy Corpsmen who train and fight with them. (In the famous photograph of Marines raising the U.S. flag on Iwo Jima in World War II, one of the six men, John Bradley, was the Navy Corpsman assigned to that platoon.)

So I chose the Navy, because Corpsman training was more extensive than the training given to medics in other branches of the military. Also, there were the beaches. I mean, c'mon—I love the sea! I didn't want to end up in the middle of nowhere a thousand miles from the ocean. All the Navy bases were on the water, on a beach somewhere, which was cool.

So I locked on to a career in the military. It was 1996, five years after Operation Desert Storm drove Saddam Hussein's Iraqi troops out of Kuwait. Saddam had been defeated, but he was still in power. It was peacetime. The Twin Towers were still part of the New York City skyline.

★★★

In the early hours of July 2, 1996, it was still dark when a Navy recruiter picked me up at my home and drove me to the airport for the flight to boot camp. I already looked the part—my good friend Tim had shaved my head several days before. I flew to the Navy's Recruit Training Command on the shore of Lake Michigan, about 30 miles north of Chicago, and began an eight-week transformation from civilian to sailor. As anyone who's been through boot camp knows, first they break you down, take away your individuality. Then they bring you back up, as a team. The whole mental game is to get the team working together. Your culture changes, your vocabulary changes, everything changes. (To this day I say "hatch" for "door" and "head" for "bathroom.")

I was okay with boot camp, but I quickly realized that not having a college degree was a major limitation. I was on the very bottom rung, looking up the ranks, at the officers, and thinking, "Man, all that guy did was go to school for four years and he gets to be an officer? I can do that." I wanted to be the officer. I wanted to be in charge. But there I was scrubbing toilets.

So I locked on to a new goal: earning a college degree. But before I could start taking courses, I had to become a Corpsman. After boot camp, I flew to the Naval School of Health Sciences in San Diego to begin my training. It was tough. I wasn't exactly the academic type in school, and suddenly I was taking classes in anatomy, physiology, and pharmacology. I had a lot of catching up to do. The pressure was on, too, because if you flunk three tests, you're outta there, back into the fleet, a regular Seaman. I was really nervous.

Of course, it wasn't all books and tests. When I wasn't studying, I was on the beach with my buddies or enjoying liberty in San Diego and Tijuana, just over the border. I was back in California, with some close buddies from boot camp. And we did everything together—PT (physical training), chow, getting into trouble, getting out of trouble. Your buddies and your group become your family.

I pulled through with decent grades and graduated as a Navy Corpsman in January 1997. Then I moved on to Camp Pendleton, north of San Diego, for three months of additional training before joining the Marines as a Fleet Marine Force Corpsman.

Some guys didn't want to go with the Marines, but I was good to go—locked on. It was awesome training. I was doing major PT, humping 12-mile patrols with gear, doing weapons training, field emergency care, land navigation, night ops—everything I needed to give me the stamina, mentality, and knowledge to support the Marines. If you're not up to that peak level, you could fail the mission.

★★★

After my training with the Marines, and for the next four years, "mission" for me was really just code for "personal goal." I plugged away toward my bachelor's degree, taking courses whenever and wherever I could. I worked in military medical clinics in California, Guam, Spain, and Hawaii. When my five years of service were up, I reenlisted for another five.

Then, in early 2001, I fell in love with a pretty Navy servicewoman named Andrea O'Malley. She knew the military and, at that point, was more decorated for service than I was. We received orders to deploy to a Navy base in Spain. We had a terrific time exploring Spain and southern France on our time off—it was an adventurous setting for our courtship! I finally popped the question on a beach in Hawaii where we were both stationed. We got married in a luau ceremony on my favorite surfing beach in the spring of 2004. Two months later, Andrea was pregnant. We found out it was a boy, and we named him Sean Patrick.

Then the word "mission" got very real, very fast. It was late summer, 2004. Operation Iraqi Freedom had stalled. A year after "shock and awe" and the toppling of Saddam's statue in Baghdad, Iraqi insurgents had reorganized and begun a series of deadly attacks using improvised explosive devices (IEDs)—bombs strapped to a body or a car and detonated to inflict maximum carnage.

The 1st Marine Division was in Iraq, and they needed Corpsmen. On our base, word went out: Corpsmen could volunteer for a seven-month deployment or they could wait to be ordered to deploy. I sat down with Andrea and we talked. We knew I'd have to go at some point because the Marines were hurting for Corpsmen. I figured that if I volunteered, I could be home for Sean's birth. It was a hard call. I wanted to be there for Andrea, of course—being pregnant is no picnic, after all. But I also wanted to do my job, do my duty, get the job done, and get home. And I wanted to be with the Marines, on the offensive. I felt it was my time to do what I'd been trained to do.

Andrea, who had already served a stint in Iraq and Kuwait, coordinating purchasing and logistics, was equally torn. She knew what it meant to serve, and she understood my desire to help out. But she was dealing with bouts of morning sickness, and afraid of what I might face in Iraq. She also had a horrible feeling about my deployment from day one. She knew I'd be with a grunt unit on the front lines. In the end, though, she agreed that I should go sooner rather than later.

My folks were worried, too. When they learned that I would need a month of combat-readiness training at the 29 Palms Marine base in the southern California desert, they decided to fly down to see me before I shipped out to Iraq. On the visit, I showed them the 14,500-pound light armored vehicles (LAVs) that were the mainstay of the Marines 3rd Light Armored Reconnaissance Battalion (3rd LAR), in which I would be embedded. I also showed them my gear and the Kevlar body armor that would protect my chest, abdomen, and groin.

My mom put on my helmet and the flak jacket. I remember her joking that there was no protection for the arms and legs. She said she wanted the knight suit—you know, a full suit of armor.

In early September, I climbed on a bus before sunrise to begin the trip to Iraq. Everybody was in full battle gear, ready to go. Most of the guys had just said goodbye to their wives or girlfriends, and children. We all carried weapons—a 9-millimeter pistol for me. It was dark outside, and dead-silent, everybody just riding with their thoughts.

★★★

After a series of flights to Kuwait, a bus convoy into Iraq, a flight on a C–130 cargo jet, and finally a helicopter flight, I landed in a tiny village in the desolate Anbar Province, hundreds of miles west of Baghdad. The Marines had established a forward operating base just outside of town. The base was little more than a handful of huts and improvised shelters surrounded by high dirt berms and guarded by short watch towers.

For the next several months I worked in the battalion aid station (BAS) where wounded Marines were brought directly from the field. Marines with minor wounds would be patched up and sent back. Those with serious injuries would be stabilized, if possible, and air-lifted to the nearest military hospital. If they needed more advanced medical attention, they would be flown to Landstuhl Regional Medical Center in Germany, the largest military hospital outside the continental United States.

When I arrived, the BAS was quiet. There were no battles going on. The Marines stationed there were mostly engaged in "hearts and minds" missions—helping rebuild infrastructure, provide security, and restore trust levels with local Iraqis.

Within the base, I was relatively safe. The danger lay beyond the berms whenever I went with the Marines on supply runs or patrols—which was often. This was at the time when the insurgents were starting to ramp up their use of IEDs. On patrols we'd vary how fast we drove to make it harder for them to time when to trigger a bomb. Everyone was constantly scanning for the trigger man.

I went along on many small-scale missions to clear specific buildings of suspected insurgents, but it wasn't until I made a supply run to a sister BAS that I encountered real casualties. I saw some Marines standing around three pairs of boots, each with an M-16 and a helmet. I knew they'd lost three buddies, but I was thinking, "That's not gonna happen to me; I'm not gonna get hurt." You start thinking about other things—training, talking to your buddies and telling stories, and you try to forget about it right away. You don't want to dwell on that stuff. You focus. You're good to go.

The next few weeks were a blur of patrols, tending to minor injuries from accidents around the base, and building bonds with the Marines under my care. I also took time to talk and sing into a portable tape recorder, sending messages to Andrea and Sean. Back in Hawaii, Andrea would listen to them and then put the speaker of the tape player on her belly, so that Sean could hear the sound of my voice.

Then rumors of a new mission began to circulate. Fallujah was heating up again. After being secured by U.S. forces and turned over to the new Iraqi army, Fallujah had disintegrated into chaos. It was now ground zero for insurgent activity. Rumor was that the United States would attack it again—soon. That would mean urban warfare, house-to-house, close-quarters fighting against an enemy impossible to distinguish from ordinary Iraqi civilians. U.S. airpower and advanced technology would help in a battle like this, but in the end the job would fall to individual Marines picking their way through a dense warren of buildings. It was the most deadly kind of warfare a Marine—or Corpsman—could face.

In the first week of November, our unit joined the most massive deployment of U.S. forces since the war had begun. Four Marine regiments and two Army regiments prepared to attack Fallujah from the north. My unit, the 3rd LAR, would attack early, from the west, both to distract the insurgents and to secure a key position: a hospital and three nearby bridges spanning the Euphrates. As I moved from western Anbar to a position just outside of Fallujah, I learned that my specific mission would be to support the Marines attempting to seize the hospital. During the fight, I would drive an unarmored ambulance—basically, a Humvee rigged with four stretchers in the back—into a live battle to pick up wounded Marines, stabilize them, and bring them back to a forward aid station. It would be dangerous as hell, but that's what Corpsmen do. It was what *I* wanted to do.

On the night of November 7th, I was at the station, waiting. It was nearly pitch-black because we had cut electricity to Fallujah. Suddenly, the sky blazed as the initial air bombardment of the city began. By the light of the rocket fire and explosions I could see that Fallujah was getting hammered.

In the predawn of November 9th, the invasion of Fallujah began in earnest with all regiments attacking from north and west. At around 10:00 A.M. the radio in the aid station crackled with an urgent request for a Corpsman and ambulance. Near the hospital several Marines from 3rd LAR had been hit with shrapnel from an exploding 82mm mortar round. This was it.

"Okay, let's go guys; we got casualties," I said.

I grabbed an M–16 and hopped into the passenger seat of the Humvee ambulance across from the driver. As we roared down the road, I had my M–16 in my right hand, sticking out the window, and the radio in my left hand. A new order came through the static: an LAV had been hit with an IED, injuring several more Marines. We were driving north, toward the Euphrates, and a line of Iraqi civilian cars had pulled to the side of the road to let us pass. Concentrating on the radio, I had no time to wonder whether the civilians were innocents or insurgents. I could see activity up ahead, and my ear was pressed against the radio. I had just turned to tell the driver to speed up when—BOOM!—we got blown up.

★★★

The IED ripped apart the Humvee and slammed my skull so hard I instantly went unconscious. I have no memory of anything that happened to me from the moment the bomb went off until about six weeks later. That doesn't mean I was in a coma that whole time. After only a few days I began to wake up for short periods; and after a couple of weeks I had periods when I was alert, aware, even chatty and humorous. But my ability to store new memories was still crippled, so all I know about that time are stories other people have told me about what I did, what

I said, and what I experienced. This section of my story, therefore, is reconstructed from their recollections, starting with an account of the immediate aftermath of the explosion, written by my captain, Matt T. Good.

According to Captain Good, the ambulance was hit on the right front side, where I was sitting, by a silver Mercedes Benz crammed with explosives. The driver of the Mercedes was killed instantly. The explosion severed my left leg above the knee, severely fractured my right foot, and sent shrapnel ripping through my arms, neck, left leg, right eye, and my mouth. The impact on my brain paralyzed the right side of my body.

From the rear of the mutilated Humvee staggered my fellow Corpsman, Ed Ronquillo. He was injured, too, and could barely walk. But seeing my leg blown open, he crawled over and applied a tourniquet, which saved my life.

"The sights and smells that I encountered as I ran up to the ambulance will be with me for the rest of my life," Captain Good wrote. "I saw Corpsman Ronquillo treating Derek's wounds. Derek was in shock. I'll never forget his eyes as he lay there. I'll never forget the cold feel of his hands and forehead as I tried to comfort him. Ronquillo was sobbing and working furiously to save him."

The battle of Fallujah raged for another two weeks and "mopping up" operations took months longer. Fifty-one U.S. service members died in the battle, and I was one of 425 who were seriously wounded. An estimated 1,200 insurgents were killed, and the operation succeeded in returning civilian governance and a sense of security to the city.

My war in Iraq was over. My war with pain was just beginning.

Ronquillo, myself, and the other wounded Marines were taken first to the forward aid station, then to Baghdad. My wounds were so severe and life-threatening that I was

immediately transferred to Landstuhl. The gravest threat
was not due to the loss of my leg, but from the injury to
my brain. As with any other tissue, the brain swells when
injured. Encased in the skull, however, the pressure from
swelling can permanently damage other parts of the brain.
If the swelling compressed my brainstem, which controls
breathing and heartbeat, I'd be dead.

Surgeons drilled a hole in my skull to relieve as much
of the pressure as possible and inserted a drain tube. They
also cleaned and sutured my many wounds as best they
could. They applied temporary treatments and dressings
to what remained of my left leg. When a limb gets blown
off in combat it's often heavily contaminated with dirt, de-
bris, and shrapnel. Closing the wound too soon increases
the risk of infection. Because it can take days for tissue
to show signs of necrosis (tissue death), they left the limb
open for the first week so that dead tissue could be surgically removed prior to closure.

While the doctors in Germany were working on me,
notification of my injuries was sent to the Naval Support
Center in Millington, Tennessee. There it fell to a Navy
Lieutenant to pick up the phone and dial Andrea's number in Hawaii.

Here's what Andrea recalls of that moment:

"It was about 4:00 A.M. Hawaii time when the phone
rang. You figure it's bad news when the phone rings in the
middle of the night, but I was hoping it was Derek calling.
The Lieutenant told me Derek had been hurt, that he'd
been hit by an IED, and that he was in Germany. I asked
him how badly Derek was wounded, but he said he didn't
have any more information."

Andrea hung up and immediately called her mother,
Kathy, in Arizona.

"I talked to my mom for a long time, and just

cried—because of course you assume the worst," Andrea recalls.

As soon as she thought someone would be in the office, Andrea drove to the base. "I walked right up to my master chief's office and said, "'Master Chief, I just got a phone call that Derek got hurt. I don't care if he doesn't come home with any legs, I just want him to come home."

Andrea returned home, and as the news spread, friends and the wives of her commanders came to be with her as she waited for more news. Meanwhile, her mother, Kathy, assuming that Andrea had called my parents with the news, called my mom, who was just getting ready for work. My mom hadn't talked to Kathy since Andrea and I were married, so she was happy to hear from her.

"I'm all cheerful and say, 'Oh, hi Kathy, how are you doing?'" my mom recalls. "And she asks me how I'm doing with the news about Derek. I say, 'What news?' So she tells me. I sat down on the floor and broke down. You break; you totally break. That's the only way I can describe it."

My mom pulled herself together enough to call a girlfriend so she wouldn't be alone—my dad was on his way to work and had no cell phone. Then she called Andrea, not only out of concern for her, but out of a powerful need to protect what might be her most tangible link to me.

This is what my mom tells me now about that call:

"This is going to sound weird," she says, "But at that point, all I knew was that you were either dead or could die. And so my main concern shifted to Andrea and Sean. I was afraid she wouldn't go to term, and then I'd have nothing. I had to help that baby. Because Sean had part of you in him."

Hours passed. Then, around noon in Hawaii, a friend of Andrea's who worked in the intelligence wing of the Army managed to find the name and phone number of the doctor in Germany who had treated me. His name was Major Mann. Andrea immediately picked up the phone. To this day she has the scrap of paper on which she furiously scribbled fragments of Major Mann's status report:

> Breathing machine
> Hit in head
> Eye surgery, drops in eyes
> Monitoring intracranial pressure
> Face peppered with burn injuries
> Shrapnel in neck
> Lower arms injured, bandaged
> Antibiotics
> Lower left leg amputated

The doctor said there was no way to tell yet how serious my brain injuries were. He also couldn't predict whether I would ever see again.

When Andrea called my mom and dad to relay the news, my older brother, Trevor, answered. He had come over as soon as he heard the news and was now fielding the calls of sympathy and support that were flooding in.

After Andrea read Trevor the list of my injuries, he said, "Hold on, I'll go tell Barb and Dave." Andrea says she heard my mom screaming in the background.

My dad vividly recalls hearing the news. "When Andrea told me about your leg, I'm thinking, well, okay, people have prosthetics. Then she talked about lacerations on your arms, and that they weren't sure if they could save your hands, and that was devastating. You can get around without your leg but you can't replace fingers."

My mom was worried about other things. "For me, it was your eyes," she says. "And the burns: I was afraid you'd be terribly scarred."

Andrea caught a red-eye to California that evening, and for the next four days they waited, getting daily updates, hoping for the best, fearing the worst. Finally they got the call that I was being transferred to the Navy's primary hospital in Bethesda, Maryland. The Navy took care of all the arrangements to fly Andrea, my mom, and my dad to Bethesda, and to set them up for an indefinite stay.

It was after midnight when they finally reached the hospital and took the elevator up to the ward where I lay. A nurse greeted them and told them I was sedated but doing okay. I was in a room with another wounded Marine, in the bed closest to the window, surrounded by a curtain.

My dad and Andrea went in first.

"I don't know if I was holding her up or if she was holding me up," my dad says. "We came around the curtain and I saw you and thought, 'He's okay—it's Derek.'"

I was lying back on a pillow, a week's growth of beard on my face and battlefield dirt still under my fingernails. I looked sunburned, with "raccoon eyes" from where my goggles had protected my skin from the blast.

"You looked much better than I thought," Andrea says. "Because the doctor had told me so many awful things about burns on your face, so I was thinking you were going to be disfigured or something, but it was just these little pepper burns. You were skinny, and your left leg was really swollen—like a foot wide. Both of your arms were bandaged up past your elbows."

There was no question by this time that my body would survive. But nobody knew if my mind, my memories, or my personality, were still intact inside my damaged brain.

★★★

For the next month, except when I was in surgery, somebody who loved me was by my bedside. Andrea's parents, Kathy and Steve O'Malley, arrived on November 16th. They took the night shift while my folks took the daytime. This allowed Andrea, now 26 weeks pregnant, to come and go as she pleased.

I soon began waking for short periods. But my entire left side remained paralyzed; I could barely see; and I was on a powerful cocktail of opioid medications, antibiotics, and anti-seizure medications. I couldn't chew or swallow solid food because my tongue had been lacerated. Many times I was utterly confused, incoherent, or agitated.

On November 18th, Andrea wrote in a diary she had begun to keep:

> Derek tried to pull his catheter out and was yanking on this drain tubes. I couldn't control him. I kept yelling "Hello!" trying to get help. He'd pull the curtains back. This was all at about midnight or so. After he calmed down, I went in the waiting room to let him sleep. Turns out he was up doing that all night. The doctors all say not to worry, that they see this every day and it's very normal. I'm scared he's going to hurt himself, especially when he kicks his injured foot against the end of the bed.

As the days passed, however, my mind slowly cleared. I recognized Andrea, my parents, Trevor, and my in-laws. I could even be funny. On November 19th, the Commandant of the Marine Corps visited me and other wounded Marines. He was a four-star general, and most people treated him with reverent dignity. I, however, was in rare form when the general came to my bedside. Here's what Andrea wrote in her journal about the scene:

> Derek was absolutely hysterical! Grinning from ear to ear! When he found out that the Commandant used to be stationed in Hawaii, he burst out with a huge smile and tells him they most definitely have to go surfing together, go do a luau, just hang out on the beach! Golf, too. The Commandant was laughing and asks Derek if he has a handicap. And Derek grins and says, "Oh yes, sir, many..." So everyone is laughing.

Those were rare moments, though. The day before Thanksgiving, I got an infection, my body swelled with fluid, and I spiked a high, dangerous fever. I was rushed to the ICU and pumped full of antibiotics. It was a close call, but the antibiotics worked, my fever cooled, and the swelling subsided.

I was also dealing with periods of intense pain. It wasn't that I was getting poor care—my relatives all praise the care I got at this time—it was simply that I was recovering from massive wounds that required frequent interventions that repeatedly stimulated my nerves. Every three days, for example, I underwent a "washout" of all my wounds and the remaining part of my left leg. This involved cleaning and removing any dead tissues. Although I felt nothing during the actual procedures, the disruption of the tissues would send massive bolts of pain shooting through my body during recovery. Even the heaviest doses of morphine were unable to dull the pain.

"You would come out of the washouts in so much pain," Andrea recalls. "I remember going with you into preop one day, and you telling me, 'Why are you doing this to me? I just want to die.' I don't think you understood what was going on. You were just in so much pain."

Most of the time the medications did control the pain, though that sometimes left me in a total fog. At one point, for example, I looked up at a nurse tending to me and I asked her if people were going to spit on me when I returned home, as some people did to returning Vietnam veterans. "No," she said, "You're a hero."

One day President Bush visited the hospital ward to personally award Purple Hearts. I did not yet have a prosthesis, and I still had metal pins in my right foot to help it heal. But I wanted to be able to stand up to shake the President's hand. I spent all morning practicing standing up, using Andrea as a crutch. A picture on the wall of my office captures that meeting: me, thin, but smiling, being held tight by Andrea while I had the honor of shaking President Bush's hand.

By early December, things were looking up. The wound on what remained of my left leg was finally closed and it had begun to heal. The doctors did not expect me to need further surgery. I also had successful surgery to repair the cornea and lenses in my right eye. Ironically, my left eye had been spared damage, but that eye had been impaired since childhood. It was my "good," right eye that took the hardest hit. Fortunately, the damage was to the outer parts of the eye, not the retina, and the doctors said they expected me to be able to see well enough to drive and to read with glasses.

Best of all, neurological testing showed that my brain was recovering well, though I would need months of physical and cognitive rehabilitation to recover lost function. Nonetheless, my short-term memory remained "broken." As I said, I can recall nothing from this period. Not the pain, not the jokes, not shaking the President's hand. It's all just a story to me.

★★★

Around Christmas time 2004, I was transferred from Bethesda to the VA Polytrauma Center in Palo Alto so that I could continue my rehab closer to home. The first memories I can recall are of being on the plane flying west with Andrea, and feeling confused. Then I remember waking up at night in the Palo Alto VA hospital, alone, and hearing the moans and cries of other patients around me. I was scared and confused because I didn't know anybody.

With increasing speed over the course of the next few weeks, my mental faculties came back "online." I had to relearn basic things, like talking, brushing my teeth, shaving, and balancing a checkbook. I also had to master new skills, such as using a wheelchair.

I now locked on to a new mission: I wanted to run again. It was an ambitious goal. It's hard for people who lose their leg *below* the knee to learn to run; but it's much more difficult for those, like me, who don't have a knee joint. I had to learn an entirely different way to run.

Obviously, before I could run, I had to learn to walk, and before that, I had to be fitted with a prosthetic. At that time, the best place in the world to get a prosthetic was Walter Reed Army Hospital, just down the street from Bethesda Naval Hospital where I initially recovered. And so, on January 11th, Andrea, who was now eight months pregnant, and I flew back east.

I began intensive physical therapy and began to use my new prosthesis. But every time I tried, I'd get shooting, stabbing pain. In an effort to alleviate my pain, the prosthetic designers created small holes in the bucketlike part of the prosthesis that fit over my remaining limb to try to reduce pressure. Still, the pain came shooting up from the tender tip of my limb. The doctors raised the dose of my medication, but that made me sleepy, and didn't stop the pain.

Then Andrea learned she had dangerously high blood pressure. The doctors recommended that she be induced early, and so, on February 15, 2005, Sean Patrick McGinnis was born at Bethesda Naval Hospital. I was there in my wheelchair, in this big room with a pullout bed for dads. Andrea did great, and it was a totally emotional moment. Sean's birth reinvigorated me to carry on. It was like, "Sean's here now, so I gotta get my life squared away. I gotta get my leg locked on."

But it was just torture. I have a very high pain threshold, but using the prosthesis was agony. I could feel something hard at the end of my limb, inside, and I thought that was what was causing my pain. My doctors were skeptical. On X-rays they couldn't see anything—just this sort of cloudy stuff. That was just *so* frustrating. I *knew* there was something going on there, so I pushed for surgery. But they kept resisting, saying I should keep working with the prosthetic. To be fair, they were frustrated, too. They seemed to have hundreds of patients scheduled into 15-minute slots and they couldn't find anything wrong with my limb. I was feeling more and more desperate. I pushed, argued, and stayed in the doctors' faces until they finally agreed to take another look—this time with a more sophisticated type of scan that gave clearer pictures of bone and soft tissues.

When the scans of my limb came back, the doctors were stunned. At the cutoff end of my left femur was a massive "bloom" of random, pathological bone growth. The medical term is *heterotrophic ossification*. The doctors said it was one of the worst cases they had ever seen.

Within a week, I was back in surgery. The ossification was cut out, the femur was cleaned up, and the limb was reclosed. Again I was told I would need no more surgeries.

Full of hope, I waited for the normal postsurgical pain to pass and for the incisions to heal so I could get into my prosthetic and resume my mission. But the pain didn't go away. It got worse. I told my doctors, "Guys, there's something extremely wrong here."

To their credit, they really did try everything—acupuncture, Botox injections, all sorts of things. Nothing worked. Now the pain was twice as bad—three times as bad—as it had been before the surgery. They wanted to raise my pain meds, but I resisted. I actually did something I shouldn't have: On my own I decided to taper down the meds. That was a mistake for a lot of reasons, not least of which because the withdrawal symptoms fueled my depression and despair.

This was when I rolled through colors on that chilly March night. I was in emotional freefall. I would cry in the shower over the futility of it all. I even told Andrea she should just leave me and find another man who would be better for her and Sean.

Fortunately—and I'll forever be grateful for this—Andrea stuck by me. She believed that I was in pain even though a social worker called her up at one point and told her he thought the pain was all in my head. Andrea also knew I was depressed and that, to some extent, this wasn't the "real" Derek. So she never even considered leaving me. On the other hand, she was getting pressure from her command to return to duty in Hawaii.

Andrea says that returning to Hawaii with Sean, knowing what bad shape I was in, was the hardest thing she's ever done. But neither of us had any choice. I had to stay in Bethesda and continue treatment. She had to do her job.

Finally, I connected with a social worker named Ansel who had been assigned to my case. He was the only guy who would listen to me. He was a straight-shooter and I bonded with him. He basically told me, "Look, they're not going to do another surgery on your leg here. They think the pain is in your head. You miss your family, so let's get you back to Hawaii. Take some liberty."

So I flew home, and for the next 30 days I relaxed around the condo, went to physical therapy, and tried to help out around the house as best I could. I couldn't wear my prosthetic, so I had to scoot up and down stairs, but I got around pretty well in the wheelchair.

The time off revived my determination to learn to run again. I began to research my options through the military's healthcare system. I discovered a new amputee care center at the Brooke Army Medical Center (BAMC) in San Antonio. I hoped that maybe there I could find a doctor who would believe my pain was real. But there was one major catch: BAMC is an Army base, which meant there was no job there for Andrea. If she wanted to join me, she'd have to get a discharge from the Navy.

Andrea had been in the Navy since 1998. She had served with distinction in Iraq, Kosovo, Thailand, and on other deployments. She was as proud of her uniform as I was and she had many longtime friends in the military. Despite all that, she says the decision wasn't hard.

"I loved Derek—we had a baby together," she says. "He was depressed—beyond depressed—and he needed me there. So I requested a hardship discharge.'"

Within a month we sold the condo and moved to San Antonio. I was under the care of Dr. Robert Granville, director of Amputee Services, who took a fresh look at my complaints. The first thing he did was use ultrasound imaging to try to see what was going on. Next, he injected an anesthetic to temporarily block a major nerve extending from my severed limb. It was both a diagnostic and thera-peutic technique—and the effect was dramatic: the pain vanished.

I was ecstatic. I was hopping around in the hallway with a big ole Kool–Aid grin on my face shouting, "I'm not a liar! I'm not a liar!"

The nerve block was only a temporary fix, however; the pain gradually returned. Fortunately, Dr. Granville didn't give up looking for a cause. Between the results of the nerve block and the imaging results, Dr. Granville suspected that my pain was related to the formation of small, misshapen pockets of fluid, called *bursa*. He was willing to perform yet another surgery to confirm his hunch and, if possible, fix the problem.

In the operating room, the problem became obvious. There *were* abnormal bursa that needed to be removed. There were also three sharp, bony spikes growing from the end of my femur, which were probably the major reason I hadn't been able to put any weight on the limb. The spikes and the bursa were removed, the femur end was again smoothed off, and the nerve that had been identified by the nerve block was severed.

This time, as the postsurgical pain faded, no new pain emerged. Within a week I could put some weight on the limb, and within a month I was in my prosthetic learning to walk. To this day I am incredibly grateful to Dr. Granville. He listened. He didn't care what the other doctors had said before. He gave me a new look, from his own perspective. If he hadn't done that and had just followed the course, I wouldn't be walking or running or doing any of the things I can now do with prostheses.

After that surgery, everything just started going up, up, up. Soon I was tackling new challenges—stairs, ramps, obstacles. I began my coursework again, did physical therapy to improve my balance, and passed the vision test that allowed me to drive again.

I also worked on the nonphysical side of my recovery. I did some one-on-one counseling, as well as group therapy with other wounded veterans. The group work was cool. We were all young, from different branches of the service, and we'd all been blow up one way or another. They'd bring in pizza, and we'd just talk. It was really helpful, because you're talking about all the stuff you've been through, and you see that you're normal. I found solace and comfort in it. We were helping each other grow back into our lives.

With things finally looking up, and me making so much progress, Andrea broached a topic that had been taken off the table during the difficult period: another child. At the time, I wasn't totally in favor of it, but after everything Andrea had done for me since the attack, I couldn't say no. Now, of course, I can't imagine *not* having another child.

Later that year, I achieved my goal: I had learned to run. I was fitted with an entirely different kind of leg from the one I use for walking. My running leg has a curving, flexible "cheetah foot," which absorbs impact and provides something like the natural spring of a foot and lower leg. Before long, I could run 5 kilometers. I began entering local races to stay motivated. I was an early member of Team Semper Fi, a group of injured Marine and Navy combat veterans who compete together in road races and triathlons.

In the summer of 2006 I locked on to a new goal: surfing. Searching the Internet, I discovered Rodney Roller, a surfer who had lost a leg in a forklift accident. Roller taught himself to surf again, went on to win several surfing competitions, and now gives clinics to other amputees. I called him up. Within a month, 12 of us wounded veterans from BAMC were on the white sands of Pismo Beach, California, on a foggy August morning, listening to Roller explain the basics of surfing. My goal was to stand up on my board within 30 minutes. A cheer went up on the beach as I succeeded, right at the 30-minute mark.

I think my passion for surfing and running and racing is partly my way of saying thank you to all the doctors and nurses and everyone who cared for me. They all used their skills so that I can walk and run, so that I can see, so that I can surf. It's almost like it's my duty not to waste what they gave me.

With the birth of Ryan, in December 2006, Andrea and I decided it was time to move closer to our families in California. We found a new single-story house in Waterford, and one of the first things I did when we moved in was to install a bracket on the front porch to hold a flag. For a while I would put the flag out every morning and take it in at night, because you're not supposed to leave a flag up overnight unless it is lighted in some way. Then I mounted a light so the flag could remain in place day and night.

Our life in Waterford is relatively simple and quiet. My brother Trevor lives the next town over with his wife and five girls. Andrea and I go to a small local church on Sundays. We take walks to the park down the street, where the boys like to chuck rocks into the Tuolumne River. Andrea keeps in shape by running and going to the gym, and she pursuing a bachelor's degree in physical education and health—a long-held dream.

In late August 2008, I drove over to nearby California State University at Stanislaus to pick up supplies I needed for my new mission: a master's degree in social work. I got my bachelor's degree in Texas, but I've decided that I want to help other veterans overcome the kinds of challenges I have faced. I work part-time for the American Pain Foundation as an "amputee advocate." I give talks (both "live" and online) about issues amputees face, and I make presentations all over the country to help build awareness of the problem of chronic pain among veterans. Once I get my master's degree, I hope to land a job in a nearby VA hospital. Until then, I try to help veterans when I can. I belong to the Waterford VFW—I'm the youngest guy there, by far. The other day an old World War II veteran came up to me and shook my hand. I had helped him file the paperwork to get him veteran's benefits. Like a lot of guys his age, he had no idea what he was entitled to.

It's now four years since I lay in the dirt, near death, on the side of a road in Fallujah. I'm grateful for all I have, and proud of the things I've accomplished. In the end, though, I don't measure how far I've come by goals achieved, or academic degrees earned, or running trophies won. For me, what counts is that pain no longer rules my life. Pain doesn't keep me from enjoying the small, ordinary moments that so many people take for granted. There's nothing sweeter than pulling into my driveway after picking up some takeout Mexican food and walking into the house, where I'm immediately tackled by Sean and Ryan. I give Andrea a hug and a kiss—she's in shorts, ready for a run. I set the food on the kitchen counter and go over to look at some drawings Sean has made. It's another hot day with near-zero humidity, and I realize we need to water three small trees we recently planted: a lemon, mandarin orange, and pear. I stand up, open the sliding glass door, grab a son in each hand, and say, "C'mon guys, let's make the trees happy."

2. Coming Home in Pain

This chapter will answer the following questions:

How many veterans have been wounded and how many are
   still in pain?
Why is coming home often so stressful for veterans?
What types of pain are veterans experiencing?
What kinds of reentry efforts—"attitude adjustments"—can
   help reduce the risk of experiencing chronic pain?
How are "wounds of the mind" related to pain from
   physical wounds?

The Price of Survival

On a sign near Camp Pendleton, painted in big letters is
the following: "The Marines are at war. America is at the
mall." That sentiment captures the wide gulf that exists
between the military and civilian worlds. More importantly, it points to one reason the experience of coming
home from war—particularly if you're wounded—can be

a whole lot different, and more difficult, than a lot of veterans expect it will be.

I've been back four years now and I still feel like an outsider—on campus, at church, around town. I just don't feel like I fit in with society, and I don't have any close friends in Waterford. I'm much more comfortable around military people, people who have shared some of my own experiences. My closest friends are the guys I run with on Team Semper Fi. They're all around the country, and we keep in touch by phone and email all the time. Most civilians simply can't understand. I'll go to a Starbucks and hear somebody who's all upset and yelling because their coffee's not right. With the perspectives that Andrea and I have gained in life, it's like, man, that's no big deal. That's what I'm talking about. If you've been at war, if you've been blow up, how can you relate to somebody who freaks out because somebody put too much cream in their frappaccino?

This kind of disconnect that veterans can experience when they get home is part of the big picture of dealing with pain. For veterans like me who were severely wounded, the transition is primarily about survival and recovery. Even for those less seriously wounded—or who are seriously hurting in less visible ways, by stress or exposure to traumatic events—the transition home can be full of unexpected complications.

The good news, of course, is that so many service men and women *are* coming home: the survival rate for those wounded in Iraq and Afghanistan is better than 90 percent. That's a medical success story that the military can be proud of and that the service members and their loved ones can be thankful for. This historically high survival rate is due to three factors, all of which played a key role in my own survival: improved body armor, surgical care deployed far forward on the battlefield, and rapid evacuation of the wounded to major hospitals on aircraft equipped with advanced life support systems. That so many service men and women survive is all the more remarkable because the wounds in Operation Iraqi Freedom (OIF) and Operation Enduring Freedom (OEF) are so often the result of bombs, not bullets—about 65 percent of the roughly 33,000 service members wounded to date were injured by IEDs, land mines, or other "blast phenomena."

The flip side of this medical triumph is an unusually high percentage of service men and women returning home from Iraq and Afghanistan in pain. For example, of the thousands of service members, like me, who are wounded by blasts, fully 60 percent suffer traumatic brain injury (TBI)—a rate much higher than in previous wars. The wounds from explosions also typically injure multiple body parts or systems, which increases the chances that the veteran will experience chronic pain of some kind. And because large numbers of Reserve and National Guard units have been deployed in these wars, the average age of service men and women has risen to 33.4 years. This, too, increases the risk for experiencing chronic pain.

Traumatic Brain Injury (TBI): Injury occurring to the brain as a result of the head violently hitting an object, or when an object pierces the skull and enters brain tissue, or when the brain is exposed to concussive blasts such as IEDs. Symptoms of a TBI can be mild, moderate, or severe, depending on the extent of the damage. Importantly, new research suggests that TBI can occur even in the absence of obvious external wounds, such as when a service member is exposed to the concussive shock waves of a nearby explosion.

Several studies have found that nearly half of all veterans seeking care from the VA report some degree of pain. Since roughly 1,350,000 men and women have served in OIF/OEF thus far, we're talking about hundreds of thousands of veterans returning home and dealing not just with the ordinary stresses of readjustment, but with the additional stress of coping with pain. The pain itself, as well as the side effects of pain treatments (such as sleepiness, sexual difficulties, or mood changes) can amplify and complicate the entire process of returning to civilian life.

Here are just some of the things that can make reentry to civilian life challenging, no matter what level of pain you may be suffering:

> ✪ **You've changed.** Military service can cause long-lasting changes in personality, temperament, and outlook. Some of those changes can be good: serving your country, putting yourself in harm's way for others, learning responsibility and discipline—these are aspects of your war experiences that can instill in you a deep sense of honor and self-respect. You may have surprised yourself by how much you accomplished in your service, which in turn may give you confidence that you can achieve other goals in civilian life. Likewise, the bonds of friendship that service members build with each other can be a source of strength and support for the rest of your life. Personally, I really enjoy going back to a base, back with "my" Marines, back to a culture I know, where I feel I'm part of something bigger than myself.
>
> Of course, there can be negative changes as well—and downsides to even some of the positive ones. For example, the emotional bonds with brothers- or sisters-

in-arms can be so deep, so strong, and so comforting that other relationships—even with a spouse—can feel shallower or less meaningful by comparison. The need to shove strong emotions, such as fear, as far into the background as possible in order to accomplish a military mission can become so ingrained that back in civilian life it becomes difficult to express—or even allow yourself to feel—emotions of any kind. Or the realities of war may change your beliefs about the value of the conflict, the validity of its goals, even your faith in government. These are just a handful of examples; the numbers of ways people change as a result of combat are as numerous as the people who serve.

✪ **Loved ones have changed.** Many service men and women are separated from their loved ones for long periods of time in both OIF and OEF, either because of multiple deployments or deployment extensions. During their time away, spouses, children, family members, and friends all continued to grow, develop, and change in response to life events. In other words, the person a service man or woman dreams of returning to may not, in fact, exist when the longed-for reunion actually happens. I was fortunate in this respect; my sons were not born when I was injured, and Andrea, being in the service herself, could understand what I was going through at a deeper level.

✪ **You're severely wounded.** Obviously, if you suffered a major wound such a head injury or one that required an amputation, you'll face many challenges when you get home. You may need to modify your home, or move altogether, to accommodate your new abilities. I remember how much work it took for my folks to adapt the bathroom when I came home for the first time, before I was using a prosthetic. And if you're seriously wounded, you'll be consumed by the demands of treatment and rehab. You may need to change career, get new training, or go back to school. In short, very little in your life will be as it was before you left.

✪ **Civilians can't understand.** War strips away many layers of culture and personality. Warriors live at the most primal level of human existence, where it is kill or be killed. Most civilians have never been the target of bullets, bombs, and mortars. They've been spared the horror of seeing a buddy killed or seriously wounded before their eyes. Neither have they been called upon to train a weapon at another human being and fire. It's more than just the brutal aspects of war that are incomprehensible to most civilians, however; the ordinary realities of military life are likewise remote from the way most civilians live. The regimentation, discipline, and command structure of the military, and the lack of privacy and freedom, are also difficult for civilians to comprehend.

> I miss all the guys. If they were all around me, piled into bunk beds, I would be laughing right now. We always laughed no matter how lousy things were. You didn't think about the bad stuff—well you thought about it just enough to make jokes about it.
>
> —*Derek McGee, former Marine gunnery sergeant in Iraq*

✪ **You miss the close contact with your friends.** Bonds of friendship formed in war are difficult to duplicate

VOICES OF SURVIVAL

For Robert Anthony, 23, returning home from Iraq was more challenging than he expected. Now studying business at Michigan State University, he says it has been difficult to make friends. "I value school more, and a lot of things in life that people our age usually take for granted," he says. "What many people find important now doesn't seem very relevant to me, like video games or who's famous."

Even common situations like sleeping in a room instead of a tent seemed weird to Anthony at first.

"It was so different," he says. "I mean, when you're used to sleeping in a tent and going to the bathroom in a port-a-potty, it was crazy just being in a room with a door. It was like you were in another world. I feel really different, in a good way and a bad way. I'm really motivated, disciplined, and I'm focused, but at the same time, it's also really hard because most people at school, they just value things differently. It's hard to explain."

Anthony returned home in pain caused by six herniated disks in his back, incurred while he was driving oil tankers from base to base, and while driving a gun truck. He also thinks he has some combat stress reactions. He says he's hyperaware of people and his surroundings, and more jumpy than he was prior to deployment. Still, he is forging on with his academic work. He doesn't want a high-powered, high-stress job, he says. Instead, he hopes to find a career that will provide some financial security but at the same time allow him to spend time with family.

For many, becoming a Marine represents one of the last all-male adventures left in America. Among them, few virtues are celebrated more than being hard—having stronger muscles, being a better fighter, being more able to withstand pain and privation. They refer to extra comforts—foam sleeping pads, sweaters, even cold medicine—as "snivel gear," and relentlessly mock those who bring it as pussies.

> —*Evan Wright, in* Generation Kill: Devil Dogs, Captain America, and the New Face of American Warfare *(New York: G.P. Putnam Sons, 2004)*

in civilian life. Not having those comrades around—the people you could tell anything to, the people you could joke with, swear with, endure hell with—can be hard.

✪ **You miss the adrenaline rush.** Although war can be terrifying, it can also be exciting—a rush. That adrenaline high just doesn't happen much in civilian life, which is why some veterans pursue extreme sports such as hang gliding, rock climbing, white-water kayaking, or motorcycle racing. The contrast between the intensity level of life in Iraq or Afghanistan and life in the United States can be disorienting.

✪ **You have no mission.** In the military, the mission is everything—and it is delivered to you in the form of orders from above. The mission is also usually crystal clear, even if the way to accomplish it is not. In civilian life, there may be no clear mission, and if there is, you usually have to generate it yourself.

✪ **There is no structure.** Once freed from the order, structure, and rigor imposed by the military, at first you may feel great, but then you may become uncomfortable. Fitting back into the workplace or classroom and the community at large can be more anxiety-provoking than you anticipate, simply because there are relatively few rules to follow compared to the military.

This short list of potential reentry stressors illustrates my point that coming home is likely to be different, and more complex, than you imagined—more emotionally complicated, stressful, and confusing. Add to that untreated or inadequately treated pain, and the reentry process becomes a high hurdle you may have trouble clearing. Severe pain may mean you can't do your job or don't enjoy recreational activities you once did. Less severe pain can still be corrosive, sapping your energy, distracting your attention, and causing you to be impatient and moody. In later chapters, you'll learn more about how pain can affect your life, as well as how you can reduce or eliminate pain. Right now, however, I want to focus on something many veterans bring home with them from war, something they may not even be aware of but which may be one of the highest barriers standing between them and getting relief from their pain: the military mind-set.

Attitude Adjustment

Military service in general, and active combat in particular, requires a host of mental armoring that protects you from harm and allows you to complete your mission. Being able to overlook discomfort and pain is one of these attitudes. Throughout basic training we are urged to "push through the pain" to reach higher levels of physical ability. Both training and deployment can involve all sorts of discomfort—freezing cold, blistering heat, blowing sand, sweat, dirt, fatigue, soreness, and exhaustion. Learning to push past discomfort, to push it into the background, perhaps even to deny that you're feeling uncomfortable, is an excellent way to adapt. On the battlefield, the "pain is not an option" attitude is an essential survival skill. The military culture encourages these attitudes and fighters who continue to shoot, continue to drive on, or—as Petty Officer Ronquillo did for me—continue to help others even when badly wounded themselves, are rightfully held up as models of heroism and dedicated service.

But macho attitudes toward pain that are useful, even healthy, in wartime, can become counterproductive and distinctly unhealthy back home. In the middle of a firefight, if you sprain your ankle, you don't stop to tape it up; you keep going and accept the risk that you might do further damage. At home, you no longer have to accept that risk. If you ignore a sprain or strain you're likely to multiply the damage, delay recovery, and increase your pain. In a war zone, a headache hardly even deserves your attention. But ignore a persistent headache at home and you may be ignoring a sign of a serious problem such as high blood pressure, chronic stress, or injury to your spine or brain—and the pain itself may seriously disrupt your work or ability to be a good parent or spouse.

My point is that when veterans come home, they need to do some serious attitude adjustment when it comes to pain, especially if they are wounded. It's just not smart or healthy to deny pain, delay seeking help, or continue on as if nothing has happened. Back home, not only is it normal to admit you are in pain, it's healthy to do so. Pain is nature's way of telling you that something is seriously wrong and requires immediate attention. Pain is not a sign of weakness. It may take some time for this to sink in, but it's essential that you leave the macho attitude behind on the battlefield.

Admitting to pain and seeking help is not just about reducing your immediate suffering—though certainly that's important. As you'll learn in more detail in the next chapter, pain can grow. Nerves carrying pain messages for long periods of time can become more sensitive to pain, which can eventually change the structure of your brain and the way you think and feel. Acknowledging that you are in pain and getting help quickly, therefore, can prevent pain from becoming "hardwired" and more difficult to treat. In addition, people in constant pain can be difficult to live with. Just ask Andrea! If you try to "tough out" the pain, you'll be adding stress to the relationships you care about and need the most. So getting help and finding ways to reduce or manage your pain is as much about looking out for others as it is about helping yourself.

> I can run to Birmingham just like this [repeat]
> I can run to Miami just like this [repeat]
> All the way to Florida just like this [repeat]
> All the way [repeat]
> Everyday [repeat)
> Ho ha [repeat]
> Suck it up [repeat]
> Blow it out [repeat]
> Suck it up [repeat]
> One, two, three, four [repeat]
> Run a little, run a little more.
> —*Marine Corps cadence*

Self-medication

Alcohol has probably been the world's oldest pain reliever. It is also the world's least effective and most

dangerous pain relief option. But because it is relatively
inexpensive and widely available, and because drinking
is historically woven into the military culture, many returning veterans turn to alcohol to escape chronic pain.
I dodged that bullet, in part, because my brain injury made drinking more hazardous than usual. I didn't
choose that path, though it was tempting, particularly
because there was a bar right next to where I was recovering at Walter Reed.

It's true that alcohol can numb pain in the short term.
But it does nothing to solve whatever physical problem
lies at the root of the pain and usually only makes the situation worse by eroding relationships, impairing your judgment and overall health, and raising your risk of having accidents,
getting into fights, and sinking into depression.

Despite these fairly well known risks, many returning service men
and women continue to drink—and often more than they did before deployment. A recent report found that Reserve and
National Guard service members who were deployed and
had combat exposure were significantly more likely to begin heavy weekly drinking and binge drinking upon their
return, compared to Reserve/National Guard members
who did not deploy.

Cutting back on your drinking, or stopping altogeth-

I shouldn't drink. I shouldn't.
My headshrinkers at the VA tell
me alcohol is not good for my
recovery, and to be honest, I have
been drinking way too much since
I got back. Self-medicating. Using
it to cover the pain, to go to sleep,
to forget, trying to fill the empty
void where my heart used to be by
crawling into a bottle. No, no, no!
Not this time, damn it.
—*Red2Alpha, Iraq veteran
and blogger*

er, can be extremely difficult, but it's certainly doable. If you think that you or someone you love is drinking to the point that they are harming their relationships, their health, or their ability to function at a job or in a family, seek help. There are many organizations and services in nearly every city and town that offer support, including independent veterans centers, where you can talk confidentially with other veterans or counselors. Check out the Resources section at the end of this book, or go to the Exit Wounds website (www.exitwoundsforveterans.org), for more information on this subject.

I don't mean to sound preachy here. I still have a glass of wine now and then—and I admit sometimes I may have a glass or two too many. The lure of alcohol for people in pain never really goes away, and it's something I still struggle with even though I avoided going down that self-destructive path early on, and am blessed in so many ways. All I want to emphasize here is to be on your guard.

Wounds of the Mind

Up to this point I've been using the word "pain" primarily to describe *physical* pain. But, of course, military personnel commonly experience many types of *mental* pain as well. Depression, grief, anxiety, posttraumatic stress, survivor guilt, and many other types of emotional distress

Survivor Guilt: A mental condition that occurs when a person perceives himself or herself to have done wrong or feels guilty because he or she survived a traumatic event. It may be found among survivors of combat, natural disaster, or life-threatening diseases such as cancer. A variant form is when a person blames himself or herself for doing too little to help those who were in danger.

can cause suffering that can be just as insidious and difficult to treat as the physical pain inflicted by shrapnel or an IED. At my lowest point, when I didn't care anymore about the flag, my service, or even my wife, I was in just as much agony as when I was suffering the bolts of pain from my physical injuries. I've seen firsthand that physical and emotional pain are intimately connected in the brain and can feed on each other. Unrelenting and unresolved pain can be deeply depressing. The depression, in turn, can make the pain worse, both directly, by disturbing normal brain chemistry, and indirectly, by making you less likely to seek help or stick to a schedule of pain-management treatments. That's why recognizing and treating the emotional wounds of war are just as important a part of your recovery mission as healing from your physical injuries.

Posttraumatic stress disorder (PTSD): A range of physical and emotional reactions that develop after exposure to one or more terrifying events that threatened or caused grave physical harm; also, witnessing harm to another person.

Posttraumatic stress disorder (PTSD), depression, and anxiety are all extremely important topics that I'll address in greater detail later. Most of this book, however focuses on physical pain, its causes and ways to relieve it. In the next chapter I'll walk you through a brief explanation of why we experience pain and how it operates in your body and in your brain. Understanding the different types of pain conditions is critical information for you or a loved one in pain; you need it to work effectively with your medical team and to advocate for the best treatment available.

THE FAMILY JOURNEY

As I said in the introduction, this book isn't just for veterans in pain. Chronic pain affects everybody involved with the person feeling the pain—especially family members. Recovery is a journey that must, therefore, include the entire family and other caring individuals. In this section and the ones like it at the end of the chapters to come, I'll suggest some ways that family members and friends can support returning veterans. These suggestions are based on my own experience, my training as a social worker, and conversations I've had with the collaborators on this book. I've also asked Andrea and my folks to contribute their thoughts about the issues raised in each chapter, because they can speak most directly about what it's like to be a spouse, family member, or friend supporting an injured service member. They have some important lessons to share!

First, here are some ways to ease the coming-home transition:

✪ Ask service members how much they want to talk about their experiences. If they don't want to talk about it, don't push. Just let them know you care about what happened, that you're willing to listen without judging, and that you want to support them.

✪ Be patient. Time can, indeed, heal, and returning veterans typically need a period to readjust to civilian life.

✪ Don't expect returning service members to be exactly as they were before they left.

✪ If a service member seems to be having trouble coping, or if you see signs of stress or inappropriate behaviors, seek professional help.

✪ Encourage returnees to connect with other veterans through local meetings, support groups, or the Internet.

✪ Refrain from raising sensitive issues if you or a loved one is tired, hungry, or intoxicated. Wait. Mornings are usually better than evenings to address emotional topics, and weekends better than weekdays.

✪ Whenever possible during conversations, use "I" statements, such as "I feel hurt when you..." or "I liked it when you..." Avoid all-or-nothing thinking that leads to expressions such as "You always..." or "You never..."

Andrea

Having someone you love come home injured and in pain is really stressful and complicated. You love them, of course, and you're so glad they're alive. But it can be exhausting, too, and confusing.

I had to make a lot of medical decisions when Derek first came back because he obviously couldn't make them himself. That was difficult because I'm his wife, and so legally I had to make the decisions, but his parents were there, too, and they cared as much about him as I did. Fortunately, we all worked together. I always asked David and Barbara before making any decision. And honestly, it brought us closer. That doesn't always happen, though. We saw a couple of really intense family arguments on the ward where Derek was recovering, which was really sad.

The most important thing you can do when a loved one comes home is to just listen to them; be as patient as you can, and don't be afraid to push back on their behalf if you don't think they're getting the care they need.

Barbara McGinnis

You need to be patient—not only with your son or daughter who is injured, but also with each other. Don't destroy your own family in the process of trying to care for your wounded service member.

I had to learn not to help Derek all the time, because he had to learn to do things himself. That's really hard for a mother! All I wanted to do was help, so I spent many hours sitting on my hands *not* doing things for Derek.

You have to defer to the spouse because they have the final say. Andrea was wonderful about always asking our opinion, but it can still be hard sometimes. As a parent, you want to say, "Hey, you've been married to him for six months, but I raised him—he's mine." You just have to bite your tongue and not say something you might regret later.

At one point, early on, we were getting really depressed about everything. We were tired, too, of

course, which made it worse. A friend of mine suggested that we try to find three things each day that
were good and focus on those. We tried it, and, by
God, it helped.

David McGinnis

We were fortunate that we could take the time
off to fly to the East Coast to be there with Derek
when he came back. I think it was incredibly important that we were there, because even though
most of the nurses and medical staff were terrific, they
couldn't do everything. We were able to pick up some
slack there. And of course, we were family, which
is probably the most important support network
any wounded veteran can have. So that's the first
thing: If you can go and be with your loved one, go.

3. The Anatomy of Pain

This chapter will answer the following questions:

How does pain work?
What are the different types of pain?
What's the difference between acute pain and chronic pain?
How can the mind or emotions affect pain?
How do conditions such as PTSD, traumatic brain injury,
     and substance abuse complicate the treatment of
     chronic pain?

Pain 101

Before I was blown up in Iraq, even with my training as a
Corpsman, I didn't give much thought to pain. As it is for
most people, pain was just something I wanted to avoid
as much as possible. That all changed when I was recovering from my injuries. Suddenly, I needed to know a whole
lot more about what pain is, where it comes from, how it
can be dealt with, and how to talk to doctors, as well as

loved ones about it. I didn't have to become a medical expert—and neither do you—but in order to be most in control of your recovery and to become an effective member of your pain management team, you have to learn at least the basics. The more you know, the better off you'll be.

For more detailed information about your particular pain disorder, check out the materials and links at the American Pain Foundation's site www.exitwoundsforveterans.org.

I find it helpful to view pain as the body's alarm system. It's a critical biological warning signal that alerts you that something is wrong with your body and triggers behaviors to avoid further damage. For instance, if your hand gets too close to a flame, the heat triggers a reflex that causes you to jerk your hand away. If your tissue is damaged, pain signals are also sent to your brain, which is where you register the pain. This is what doctors call **acute pain**. It can be caused by such things as an injury, infection, or surgical procedure. Acute pain typically lasts only a matter of hours or, at most, days, and it fades as healing proceeds.

If pain remains even after an injury, infection, or surgery has healed, or if it simply continues for longer than expected, it's called **chronic pain**. About 76 million people suffer from this kind of pain in the United States alone, and it's the type of pain I experienced for so many months. Chronic pain is debilitating, frustrating, and exhausting. It becomes the focus of your entire life. Work, play, and relationships all suffer.

Chronic pain may be due to some type of continuing tissue injury, such as arthritis, a pinched or damaged nerve, or constant muscle spasms. Other times the tissue has healed, but the pain continues. In these cases, the pain "alarm system" may be broken. The pain signals are real, but they no longer serve as a warning of injury or illness; rather, they are generated by the nerves themselves, which have become damaged or hypersensitive. Pain that arises even when there is no danger of harm may be called chronic pain. It's important to appreciate the difference between acute and chronic pain because the two types respond differently to pain treatments, such as medications or nerve blocks. (I'll talk about these and all the other types of treatment options for pain later in the book).

Unlike acute pain, chronic pain may get worse with time. When nerves continuously fire off pain signals, they produce a number of chemicals that make the nerves more sensitive, more likely to send even more pain signals. This results in a condition called hyperalgesia. You can see how this situation can become a vicious circle: pain produces sensitization, which produces more pain, which produces more sensitization, and on and on. A related condition is neuropathic pain, which is a type of chronic pain caused by alteration of the nervous system involving damaged or malfunctioning nerves. The takeaway point for veterans is that getting help for your pain quickly can reduce your risk of suffering from chronic pain.

Acute pain occurs suddenly due to illness, injury, or surgery. It doesn't last long and subsides as injured tissue heals.
Chronic pain persists for long periods of time (usually three months or more) and continues even after a wound has healed.
Neuropathic pain is a type of chronic pain caused by damaged or malfunctioning nerves. Unlike acute pain, it may get worse as time goes on.
Hyperalgesia is an increased sensitivity to pain, which may be caused by damage to pain receptors or nerves that carry pain signals.

Measuring Pain

One of the most problematic aspects of pain, whether acute or chronic, is that it can't be measured with any kind of blood test, sensor, or scan. Being told, both directly and indirectly, that my pain was "all in my head" illustrates the point. It sure as hell was *not* all in my head but I couldn't prove it.

That said, pain is subjective, meaning that doctors must rely on their observations of your behavior (for instance, when I'd shout in pain when I tried to stand in my prosthetic) and what you *tell* them you are experiencing. Despite my experience several years ago with one or two doctors who didn't believe me, the fact is that more and more doctors are accepting the maxim that *pain is what the patient says it is.* Increasingly, doctors and other healthcare professionals are adopting the attitude that patients are being honest and as accurate as they can be in reporting what they are feeling. Fortunately, these days, you shouldn't have to look too far to find a doctor who will take your pain seriously—as Dr. Granville did with mine. In fact, there is growing appreciation within the medical community that pain should be considered the "fifth vital sign"—to be checked and taken as seriously as the traditional four vital signs of blood pressure, pulse, respiration, and temperature. Vital signs have historically given healthcare providers important clues to diagnose and treat illness. Pain is now being recognized as providing a useful tool for providers to measure and monitor a patient's state of health, illness, and well-being.

Pain scales allow healthcare workers to assess the relative severity of the pain a patient is experiencing. By using a pain scale over time, a patient can see more clearly if their pain is getting better or worse.

Even though pain cannot be seen on an X ray, there *are* ways to measure or describe a person's subjective experience of pain. For example, if you come to a doctor in pain, one of the first things you'll be asked is to describe, as specifically as possible, exactly how the pain feels. At first this seems almost silly to some people. They're likely to respond, "I don't know...it just *hurts!*" That's understandable, but not very helpful. The fact is that pain comes in many "colors." It can be sharp, dull, burning, shooting, throbbing, easy to locate or diffuse, to name just a few of the ways it can be described. Being specific about how your pain feels can provide important clues to doctors about what's going wrong in your body to cause the pain.

You may also be asked say how intense your pain feels. Doctors often gauge pain intensity with a **pain scale** that ranges from 0 (no pain) to 10 (worst imaginable pain). Another type of scale uses cartoon-like faces to express varying pain intensities. I found that putting a number on my pain—even if it was an excruciating 10—gave me a sense of control and a handle on something that otherwise seemed totally out of control and crazy.

Another tool for assessing and tracking your pain over time is a pain notebook. (One is available free from the APF website, at www.painfoundation.org) A pain notebook can help you record details of your pain experience (e.g., when it occurs, for how long, the level and type of pain, possible triggers, etc.), its impact on your day-to-day life (e.g., activities you can or cannot do), and how you respond to various treatments over time (e.g., side effects and improvements in daily function and emotional wellness). By noting what makes your pain better or worse you can help your healthcare team find the best treatment approach for you. Plus, you'll be playing a more active role in your care, which can go a long way toward helping you stay positive and feel in control.

The Phantom

One type of pain deserves special mention in this book: **phantom pain.** In 1551, French military surgeon Ambroise Paré wrote that, "Patients, long after the amputation is made, say that they still feel pain in the amputated part." More than 300 years later, another military surgeon coined the term "phantom limb" to describe this phenomenon. In 1871, Civil War physician Silas Weir Mitchell wrote that "thousands of spirit limbs were haunting as many good soldiers, every now and then tormenting them."

The reason people with amputations often have the vivid sensation that a missing limb or body part is still there (called **phantom sensation**) or experience sharp pain in a missing limb, is that the brain contains a detailed map of the entire body. This neural map, or model, remains even though a limb or other body part is gone. And if the nerves connected to that map misfire, you will have the very odd experience that the limb or body part is still in place.

I've experienced both phantom sensations and phantom pain. Phantom sensation is just plain weird. You know it's in your head, but it feels so real. Even right now, sitting here, I have a tingling in my missing left foot, and I have the sense I'm wiggling my nonexistent toes in an effort to make it go away. My toes feel as if they're in wet concrete as I do so. What I'm doing is using my mind to move nonexistent body parts to curb the sensation from a nonexistent body part. Like I said:

Phantom pain: A type of neuropathic pain that results in feelings of pain in a nonexistent body part.
Phantom sensation: The vivid awareness of a nonexistent body part, which may or may not be accompanied by cramping, tingling, or other sensations that fall short of actual pain.

VOICES OF SURVIVAL

I was in Vietnam with Special Forces, and we were jumping from a C-130. The man before me stepped off, rather than jumping, and his static line didn't rise far enough. It caught across my throat when I jumped and I got tangled in the static line. I was bouncing against the side of the plane, when someone in the plane cut the static line holding me. The people in the plane thought I was probably dead, but my static line opened my chute. I came to when I was about 300 feet from the ground. I had just enough time to drop my pack before hitting the ground on top of my pack.

I hurt from the beating I took from bouncing against the aircraft. I also had burns across my throat from sliding down the static line. Even though I felt like I had been run over by a truck, I got up, collapsed and stowed my chute in the bag, put my pack on, flipped the bag with my chute over my head, and walked off the DZ. A little pain wasn't going to stop me.

Two days later, I couldn't move. I was in so much pain I couldn't describe it. They put me in the hospital and gave me morphine. The Army then shipped me stateside. A year later I was discharged from the Army, and that is when the VA started treating me.

I was in agonizing pain. The VA awarded me a 30 percent disability. I had a wife and two young kids, so there was no question that I had to go back to work. Back strain was the official name of my injury until 2000, when I finally found out the medical name for my disease. All I knew was that I was in intractable pain all of the time. I had sciatica down both legs; my hands hurt; and my hands and arms were numb from the elbow down.

(continued)

weird.
(*Voices of Survival continued*)

After years of treatments that didn't work, I went back
to the VA and they ran more MRIs. The neurosurgeon
told me I had arachnoiditis (inflammation of one of the
membranes surrounding the brain and spinal cord). Today,
my disability is rated 100 percent service-connected,
effective June 2001. The pain clinic has put me on the
Duragesic patch, which controls my pain. But before they
gave me the patch they tried various opiates: morphine,
methadone, tramadol. None of them worked. I threw up
a lot. I lost 40 pounds looking for a medication I could
tolerate. The patch, combined with other medications to
treat pain, has given me a great deal of relief from my pain.

My life was changed on that day in Vietnam, but I
never gave into my pain. I work full-time and always have.
I own a real estate company and a mortgage company. I will
never let my pain control me. It is too easy to submit to pain
and allow it to control your life. I will never stop fighting.
                    —Posted by Stephen on the American Pain
                    Foundation website

Phantom pain is different—and a lot worse. Initially,
I had extreme phantom pain in my third, fourth, and fifth
toes. Sometimes, it felt like they were cramped under-
neath my foot, and it was excruciating. I also sometimes
got jolts of pain that would shoot up my leg. I'm happy
to report that by using a variety of techniques, which I'll
discuss in Chapter 6, I now only rarely have phantom
pain—though I still have phantom sensations and probably always will.

The Long Arm of Pain

I want to end this brief overview of pain by reminding you how tightly connected pain is with every other aspect of your life. Pain isn't just a problem with one part of your body or with a set of damaged nerves. Think of the alarm analogy again. Imagine trying to carry on your life with an alarm bell ringing inside your head that you can't shut off. Yes, the fundamental problem is with the alarm itself, but that unstoppable clanging means you can't concentrate or appreciate anything else—not your work, your spouse, your kids, or any other aspect of normal life. This can lead to other problems, such as depression, alcoholism, and substance abuse.

Unfortunately, the relationship between pain and these kinds of life problems is a two-way street. Untreated or under-treated chronic pain may lead to harmful coping strategies such as substance abuse. But drinking or using other kinds of drugs is very likely to make the pain *worse*, not only because of rebound reactions after the drug has worn off, but because heavy drug and alcohol use gets in the way of the work you need to do to take control of the pain, find an effective treatment, and stick to it. That's just one example. For veterans, the problem can be compounded by posttraumatic stress disorder (PTSD) and traumatic brain injury (TBI). Any one of these conditions will complicate, and potentially worsen, any pain you may be suffering. Having more than one—which is fairly common—makes this more challenging, but still doable.

The tightly-woven connection between pain and other aspects of your life is why pain is best fought on many fronts. It's never enough to focus just on pain relief. If there are other serious issues in your life such as substance abuse, depression, or PTSD, you must address these as well. In fact, sometimes you must make progress on these problems *before* pursuing direct treatment of chronic pain.

In this chapter I've tried to give you a crash course in pain. You saw that some types of pain feel different from others, and that pain may be acute or chronic (and possibly neuropathic). You also learned that pain can intensify because nerves that are constantly firing off pain signals can grow more sensitive over time. We took a look at phantom sensation and phantom pain, which affect thousands of veterans today. Finally, you saw that untreated pain can both cause and be amplified by other life problems such as depression and alcoholism. The good news is that many treatments are available today to treat chronic pain, in all its guises. Before I turn to those subjects, however, it's important to take a closer look at the many ways that pain can affect the life of a returning veteran, which is the subject of the next chapter.

THE FAMILY JOURNEY

As a Navy Corpsman, I knew a fair amount about how pain works and how it can be relieved. But once I was injured and became a patient in pain, that wasn't enough. I was torn up physically, mentally, and emotionally. At first, I couldn't even speak. That meant my family members needed to learn about pain, too, and I needed their help to stay on top of my medical treatments and make choices about treatment options. Recovering from chronic pain required organization, morale-boosting, and self-advocacy and self-education. If you're lucky enough to have family around to be part of your medical support team, make good use of them. Don't worry about being a burden to them, and don't try to tough it out on your own. You know from your training that you have to rely on others during a mission. It's the same during recovery. Accept help wherever it comes from—you can make it up to them when you've healed.

My advice to family members is to learn as much as you can about the condition of an injured service member, and don't be afraid to ask questions until you fully understand the situation.

Here are some other ways that family members might help somebody experiencing chronic pain:

✪ Encourage them to seek help sooner rather than later to reduce the risk that their pain will get worse or become "hardwired."

✪ Accompany them on doctor visits, both to provide moral support and to act as a second pair of ears taking in the information being given.

✪ Take notes during doctor visits.

✪ If a doctor seems to be dismissing a loved one's pain, or suggests that it's "all in their head" urge him or her to find another doctor.

✪ Encourage a service member in pain to build a team of providers rather than relying on just a family physician or any one medical professional.

✪ Encourage a person in pain to find a pain specialist or other healthcare provider who can introduce ways to harness the power of the mind to help control pain.

Andrea

If your partner isn't taking care of the pain, you may have to push them to make appointments, or even make appointments for them, especially if you have a partner who doesn't like to make phone calls or take the time to do stuff like that. I don't have that problem with Derek because he's a good advocate for himself, but I know some spouses do.

In the end, your spouse has to be the one who wants to get help—you can't do it for them. All you can do is remind them, let them know what their options are, and urge them to keep pushing and not give up.

Barbara McGinnis

Sometimes Derek wanted to get off his pain medications too quickly. He'd call and I'd say, "Honey, I think you need to stay on a little bit longer." So you try to encourage them and say what you think, but, of course, it's their decision in the end. You have to let go of your children at some point. You're still involved, of course, but you have to almost treat them as a friend.

4. The Consequences of Untreated Chronic Pain

This chapter will answer the following questions:

How does chronic pain add to the sense of isolation felt by
many veterans?

How are family members, spouses, children, and others
affected by a service member's pain?

In what ways does pain interfere with your work, career, or
education?

How does chronic pain increase your risk for depression
and suicide?

The Truth about Consequences

For service members such as myself who have been seriously wounded in combat, it's not hard to see how our
injuries affect our lives back home, especially in the early
phases of recovery and adaptation. But there can be fairly serious consequences even for service members who
haven't lost a limb, sustained brain injury, or suffered

some other kind of severe injury. Many service members either sustain less traumatic wounds or return home with back problems, joint problems, or other type of ailments that are not considered "wounds" at all. But all types of wounds can make it harder to readjust to work and family life, particularly if chronic pain is involved.

In this chapter I want to spend some time talking about the dangers of untreated chronic pain because I think many returning veterans and their family members may not fully grasp just how serious this situation can be. I'm not just talking about the dangers of the pain getting worse—though as you saw in the previous chapter, that's a real concern.

Some of the wounded soldiers I've been working with do not get the pain care they need because they are afraid to ask for it, are ashamed to ask for drugs to control their pain due to social stigmas associated with the abuse of pain medications, or are simply trying to be tough. The fear of addiction and the associated stigma of drug use, ironically, may lead to more profoundly addictive behavior. One of my old soldiers was wounded and returned from Iraq this past summer. As we were talking, he bragged that he was not using his pain meds; but unfortunately it turns out, he was self-medicating with alcohol to cope with the pain.

—*Captain Jonathan D. Pruden, U.S. Army, testimony at the Congressional Hearing on Chronic Pain, December 8, 2005*

I'm talking about all of the nonphysical consequences of chronic pain—and there are a lot of them! Here's a list of the more serious potential hazards:

- ✪ Isolation
- ✪ Substance abuse
- ✪ Physical deconditioning

- ✪ Sleep disturbance
- ✪ Reduced sexual activity
- ✪ Family stress
- ✪ Impaired ability to work
- ✪ Lowered self-esteem
- ✪ Irritability
- ✪ Depression

I talk about these consequences not to belabor the problems, and certainly not to bum you out. All of the challenges I discuss below *can be managed* in one way or another. None of these consequences is a dead end, as you'll learn in later chapters when I describe ways to cope with them. My goal here is to emphasize the seriousness of this condition for those who might be tempted to try to "tough it out," or for those who are not aware of how drastically chronic pain can affect their life. I hope that by going into some detail about these consequences—and quoting extensively from those who have suffered—you, too, will learn to take your pain seriously, seek help sooner rather than later, and not be afraid to admit you are in pain. As you'll see below, the stakes of not doing so are very high!

Isolation

Nature has designed pain to be hard to ignore. As I said in Chapter 3, pain is the body's alarm system, and when it goes off, it typically trumps everything else in your life. Your social life is often the first casualty as you rush to respond to the wail of pain's siren. Bowling? Forget it. Dancing? No way. Even going to a movie can hurt and,

There are days when I feel like a broken bottle; all the pieces hurt, and I can't seem to bring them together to make an entire vessel. Sleepless nights, days where you don't want to see anyone, do anything, or go anywhere.

—Anonymous post #6 on the American Pain Foundation website

therefore, not seem worth the effort.

Returning veterans may, of course, feel socially isolated even without pain in their lives, for all of the reasons I discussed in Chapter 2, but chronic pain makes the challenge of reentry even tougher. It makes it harder to connect with friends, family, and co-workers, and sets the stage for unhealthy ways of coping with isolation, such as by drinking or using drugs.

Substance Abuse

In classic western films, whisky is the all-purpose anesthesia. Need to remove an arrow? No problem, give the guy a few slugs and yank. Sterilize a wound? Pour whisky on it! Want to forget that gal who ditched you back in Dodge City? Reach for that hip flask while sitting by the camp fire and drown your sorrow.

In real life, it's not much different: many people in chronic pain use alcohol or other drugs such as cannabis to self-medicate. For veterans, the pull of drugs can be very strong. Drinking, for example, is an ingrained part of military culture. And alcohol can ease pain, at least temporarily, because it depresses the central nervous system, slows brain function, and provides a fuzzy sort of relief.

Alcohol, however, is also an extremely hazardous drug, and more so for people returning from military duty and in the midst of coping with the stresses and strains of readjustment. I don't think I need to list the ways alcohol can hurt you or your loved ones—we're all grown-ups here. Most people who drink already know it will make them quicker to anger, more likely to get into fights or give way to depression, and become a danger behind the wheel; they also know they're likely to feel worse, not better, the next morning.

Still, it's worth emphasizing here that using alcohol to excess will almost always make everything worse—your ability to cope, to be in a relationship, to work, to be a good parent—everything. And if you are taking some kind of pain medication—which is the case for most people in chronic pain the combination is *potentially lethal.* Alcohol can dramatically *enhance the sedative effects of many types of pain medications, making the combination potentially lethal.* And even for people who think they "know their limits" with alcohol from years of experience, the addition of pain medications makes that experience irrelevant and can lead to very risky behaviors while under the influence, including driving, using a firearm, or operating dangerous machinery.

I don't want to sound like your mother here. And as I've said before, it's not like I don't drink or feel tempted sometimes by the bottle. I'm doing okay and

Most nights when Anthony Klecker, a former Marine, finally slept, he found himself back on the battlefields of Iraq. He would awake in a panic and struggle futilely to return to sleep. Desperate for relief, Mr. Klecker, 30, drank heavily. One morning, his parents found him in the driveway slumped over the wheel of his car, the door wide open, wipers scraping back and forth. Another time, they found him curled in a fetal position in his closet.

—*Lizette Alvarez, "After the Battle, Fighting the Bottle at Home,"* New York Times, *July 8, 2008*

Roughly 10 percent of the general population is at risk for becoming addicted to drugs, alcohol, or other types of addictive behaviors such as compulsive gambling. This predisposition has complex roots in both genetics and upbringing. Until an individual is exposed to alcohol, drugs, or potentially compulsive activities, however, it's difficult to know if they are among those with an inborn vulnerability to addiction.

things are under control. But I'm not above temptation and I know from personal experience that everything's different when you're in pain. We human beings have a well-honed ability to deceive ourselves about our own capabilities and to deny our problems. If you take a hard look at how much you're drinking, and you think it's too much, it probably is. Cut back, stop, or, if you can't stop on your own, get help.

Physical Deconditioning

The service men and women who make it through the various boot camps are at the peak of physical conditioning. In all branches of the military, PT is a central, constant element of life. Being lean, "buff," and strong is a source of pride and satisfaction for many military men and women—myself and my wife Andrea included. That's why it can be particularly cruel when chronic pain prevents us from maintaining our conditioning. Many men and women will tolerate a huge amount of pain to keep running, keep training, keep lifting weights, keep doing reps; but chronic pain can conquer the strongest will. When it does, an inevitable result is physical deconditioning—a loss of muscle tone and mass and an increase in fat deposits. This can be a wrenching and depressing situation for many OIF/OEF veterans, and it's often a strong motivation to seek professional help.

Exercise is such an important part of any recovery program that I devote all of Chapter 7 to it. For now, I just want to stress that physical deconditioning is another potential consequence of chronic pain, one that can be very important for service members.

Sleep Disruption

Many people aren't aware of this fact, but sleep is one of the most vital components of healing; and because chronic pain disrupts sleep, it impairs one of its key remedies. Roughly 70 percent of veterans of OIF/OEF who report some kind of painful condition also say they have poor or unrefreshing sleep. That's a big deal. The value of sleep to people's overall mental and physical health is greatly underappreciated. Most people get less sleep than they should, and they compensate with caffeine or other stimulants, which usually just makes it harder to sleep the following evening.

Those in pain often are all too aware they're not getting enough sleep—they can't get comfortable, and they toss and turn all night. Sometimes, however, the problem isn't so obvious. People normally cycle through stages of sleep, including periods

> Even just walking hurt. As someone who had run, played ball, biked, chain-sawed, or did something else strenuous every day of my adult life, it was troubling to find that a flight of steps wiped me out. Climbing steps took gripping both hands on the railing, hard, rising one stair at a time.
>
> —*Bob Nylen, Army veteran, from post on the APF website*

called "micro arousals" when they emerge naturally into a light, non-dreaming state of sleep that doesn't have the healing benefits of deep sleep. Pain can lead to many more of these micro arousals. People in pain may not realize they have spent much less time in deep, healing sleep; they may know only that they wake up not feeling as refreshed or ready for the day as they used to.

The problem of sleep deprivation is complicated by the use of pain medications, which can profoundly alter sleep rhythms. Alcohol, too, can disrupt sleep, by promoting drowsiness early in the evening then producing "rebound" wakefulness in the middle of the night as the sedative effect of the alcohol wears off. For service members dealing with combat stress issues or diagnosed PTSD, having frequent nightmares can also destroy a good night's sleep.

Bottom line? Sleep disorders are a huge problem even for veterans who are not physically wounded, and it's an even bigger problem when a returning service man or woman is battling chronic pain.

Reduced Sexual Activity

Sadly, one of the first things to disappear from the life of somebody in chronic pain is an activity that is actually fairly good at relieving pain: sex. The relaxation, emotional tenderness, comfort, and release of endorphins typically accompanying sex all reduce pain. The irony is that if you're in pain—especially if it's pain caused by moving parts of the body involved in sex, such as the back and pelvis—making love may be the last thing you're interested in.

Pain can impair your sex life in many ways. Either you or your partner may be afraid of causing more pain by engaging in lovemaking. The person in pain may not feel very attractive or sexy, or may not have the energy or motivation to pursue sex. On top of these barriers, many pain medications can interfere with sex drive, the ability to get an erection, and/or the ability to have an orgasm.

For many people, intimacy issues are easier to ignore than to deal with head on. Like most problems we'd rather push under the rug, however, not dealing with sexual issues takes its toll on individuals, on couples, and on marriage. In Chapter 8, I'll talk more about how and where to get help if this has become a problem area in your life.

Before I deployed down range, I was different about my wife and kids. Now that I'm back I can only let them get so close before I have to get away from them. I used to have fun letting my boys jump and crawl all over me. We would spend hours playing like that. Now I can only take a couple of minutes of it before I have to get out. I usually get in my truck and drive back to the base to be with my platoon.

—*Paratrooper home from Iraq, quoted in* Down Range: To Iraq and Back *by Bridget C.Cantrell and Chuck Dean (Seattle, WA: WordSmith Books, 2005)*

Family Stress

Living with somebody in chronic pain isn't as bad as being in pain yourself, but it's no picnic either. Just ask my wife, Andrea! A spouse, children, parents, or other companions may have to pick up a lot of slack around the house because a service member can't lift, move easily, drive, or do other basic tasks. Frustrations can build on both sides. The one in pain may feel guilty or sad that he or she can't help, as in the past. The person doing the supporting may feel unfairly burdened or irritated, but at the same time not want to say anything because he or she knows how much pain the returned veteran is feeling. The result can be a real stew of complicated, conflicting emotions. Fights, tension, and unresolved or unacknowledged hostility between spouses or partners can be a major contributor to the overall stress a person in chronic pain is feeling.

Inability to Work

Whether you're a bricklayer or an accountant, chronic pain is likely to disrupt your work. Certainly, chronic pain can prevent you from doing physical tasks such as lifting, bending, or carrying heavy objects. Similarly, the gnawing irritation of chronic pain can make it difficult to concentrate on purely mental tasks such as writing, programming, computation, or analysis. And if the pain itself isn't disruptive, the medications used to treat it may be—which is another good reason to be persistent and assertive in your search for a treatment that not only relieves your pain but improves your ability to function at home and work.

> I never got to enter that world of professionals because it's hard to work when you're hurting all of the time, and employers don't want to hear you telling them, "I'm in too much pain to work today."
>
> —*Afi, posted on the American Pain Foundation's "Voices of Pain" website*

Lowered Self-esteem

Cynthia's quote here pretty much says it all: being stripped by chronic pain of your ability to function normally can really take a chunk out of your self-esteem. You may feel humiliated by your helplessness and frustrated that you even feel that way because, of course, your head "knows" you are doing the best you can.

Chronic pain can also lead to the loss of other sources of self-esteem, such as your job, your role as breadwinner, your athletic abilities, or your role as a leader in community organizations. Losing your self-esteem can be as devastating as losing a limb—and there's no prosthetic for it! You have to build it back yourself, piece by piece. I'm living proof that some people with serious wounds and chronic pain can recover their function—and their self-esteem—with proper treatment.

> I cannot lift so much as a gallon of milk or brush out my own hair; and on high pain days, I cannot properly dress myself. I am ashamed at how little I can do following this travesty. I am a very proud person who is humiliated by the life I am forced to lead.
>
> —*Cynthia, post on the American Pain Foundation website*

Irritability

People naturally become more irritable, short-tempered, and grouchy when they're tense, tired, hungry, or all of the above. No surprise, then, that chronic pain can cause a quantum leap in a person's level of irritability. The simple fact of having pain that isn't being relieved is frustrating and irritating;

> You're having the time of your life, and from out of nowhere, you're stopped by the most terrible pain you've ever felt in your life. Your lower back is hurting so bad you have no choice but to cry in pain! It takes all you have to roll over. And your girlfriend/lover/wife asks you, "Are you okay?" And you want to get mad as a hornet. But you can't. You're finished.
>
> —*Posting by chronic pain sufferer on APF website*

add to that the effects of interrupted sleep, the stress of not being able to do a job or enjoy recreational activities, and the mood-altering effects of pain medications, and you have all the ingredients for a "perfect storm" of foul temper!

Depression

Pain and depression are tightly linked: pain causes depression; depression causes (or amplifies) pain. Roughly one out of every three patients with persistent pain suffers from clinical depression related to that pain, and almost all persons in chronic pain will experience some mood changes; 75 percent of patients with clinical depression come to their doctors complaining of physical symptoms, including pain. People in pain who are also depressed experience greater impairment than those who aren't depressed.

Depression and pain go hand in hand for a lot of reasons. One is that both mood and pain signals are affected by the same kinds of brain chemicals—neurotransmitters—such as dopamine, serotonin, and norepinephrine. In addition, high levels of stress

It was Thanksgiving. I was at my grandparents house; lots of aunts and uncles and cousins around. At the top of the hour, CNN gave the highlights of another day in Iraq, in Baghdad. Tens and tens killed and hundreds wounded in Sadr City by IEDs; hospitals packed with wounded, flooding into hallways awash in blood. I snapped: "Can we please watch something else for fuck's sake?!" I might as well have taken a shit on the living room floor. All conversation stopped and everyone looked at me as I stood there frozen. Not knowing what to do, I stormed out of the room to the bedroom I was staying in.

—*Red2Alpha, Iraqi veteran and blogger, from www.soldierlife.com*

hormones, particularly cortisol, have been linked to depression. Chronic pain itself can raise cortisol levels, and being in combat situations does the same thing, even if you aren't physically wounded. When your brain is constantly bathed in stress hormones, you may be more susceptible to depression and chronic pain symptoms later in life.

Interestingly—and encouragingly—some of the same medications used to treat depression also help reduce chronic pain. Again, this is because many similar brain regions and neurotransmitter systems are involved in the two disorders. I'll be talking more about the issue of depression in later chapters. Here, I just want to restate the seriousness of depression because of its most tragic possible outcome: suicide. As I mentioned in the introduction, the current rate of suicide among OIF/OEF service men and women is the highest since these statistics began being kept, in 1980. This is not simply due to high levels of chronic pain. Other factors are at work, including the higher-than-normal levels of PTSD among these veterans, the complexity of the wounds suffered by OIF/OEF veterans, and the increased likelihood they'll face some kind of pain they can't control.

> After a stay in the hospital and a year of physical therapy, the doctors said they could do no more for me, that I would have to learn to live with the pain. It was such a blow; I thought that they could fix me and my life could go on. What a shattering blow to find out that you will never be the same again. That triggered my first suicide attempt.
>
> —*Anonymous post #7 on the American Pain Foundation website*

Neurotransmitter: A chemical in the body that carries information between nerve cells. Different kinds of neurotransmitters carry different types of messages from one nerve cell to another.

Moving Forward

Throughout this chapter, I've been talking about all of these possible consequences of chronic pain as though they are separate from one another. But, of course, they're not. Life is difficult, and many of the symptoms of chronic pain blur and bleed into each one another. A good example is depression, which can lead to drinking, which can deepen the depression and the experience of pain, which can result in the breakup of a relationship, which can lead to more depression. You get the picture.

Fortunately, there is a good-news side to this equation. *If you can improve one area in your life, other areas may improve as well.* Yes, it's possible to get caught in a self-perpetuating downward spiral. But it's equally possible to create a self-reinforcing *upward* spiral. The most obvious way to start is by getting competent, professional, and comprehensive help for your chronic pain condition. As you will learn in the next chapter, the goal of treatment is to *improve your function* in all areas of your life. If that can be done—and it can almost always be done if you stick with it—then the upward spiral can begin. You might be able to return to work, for example, which can raise your self-esteem, reduce family tension, and ease depression—all of which will help to further reduce your pain.

The key is to begin—though that doesn't necessarily mean attacking the pain condition immediately. If somebody is suffering from alcoholism, he or she may need to enter rehab and recover before real progress can be made. Same goes for depression: a depressed person will not have the energy or motivation he or she needs to stick to a program of pain management. He or she may need to get prompt treatment for the depression before making progress on the pain front, or at least pursue treatments simultaneously.

There simply is no one-size-fits-all answer here. You, with the help of your healthcare providers and, I hope, an experienced pain specialist, will create a road-map for recovery, one tailored to your specific needs and priorities.

THE FAMILY JOURNEY

This chapter touches on some big issues. Depression alone is an enormous topic—entire books have been written about it. I want to focus here on some concrete things you as a family member can do if you see that someone you love is suffering from one or more consequences of chronic pain.

✪ Keep the lines of communication open. Talk about issues and concerns as they arise. Remember that "revealing is healing."

✪ Be as patient as possible with a family member's limitations without becoming an enabler of helplessness. Trust your instincts about when to help and when to encourage self-help.

✪ Listen without trying to fix or solve an issue or problem.

✪ Encourage some kind of physical activity every day, even if it is very small. Even people in severe pain can usually move to some extent, or move some part of their body. Doing even very small range-of-motion exercises can be helpful and can provide a way to measure progress.

✪ Take care of yourself.

✪ Look for support groups dealing with the same issues you are. Support groups for care providers, spouses of veterans, spouses of people dealing with substance abuse, and many others are available. (See the resources section at the back of this book for a short list, and the Exit Wounds website for a complete list of places to find such groups.)

✪ Learn more about the specific problem a service member might be having (e.g., sleep disorders, depression, or sexual problems) by reading, talking to others, or consulting with a family healthcare provider.

Andrea

I think people really need to trust their instincts. If you sense there is a problem with a relationship, or that something's going on with a person you love, there probably is a problem.

If you see your partner having a problem, you've got to say something. It's sensitive—you don't want to say something that makes the person get totally defensive. I didn't have to do that much with Derek, but I did a couple of times. I remember when we were in San Antonio and he was still recovering from his brain injury. He was having lots of memory problems and I felt he needed more brain rehab. We'd lived there three months and he still didn't remember our phone number, and he'd ask me for it all the time and it was starting to get a little annoying. So I said, "I really think you should get some help with this." And he listened to me. He didn't take anything personally.

Barbara McGinnis

You know, it's not just the veterans who can get into trouble with alcohol. Parents need to be careful, too. We're social drinkers, and alcohol isn't a problem for us, but I remember as we were flying to Bethesda that first time, Dave turned to me and said, "Let's not start drinking, because I'm afraid we'll never stop." And we didn't—we didn't drink at all during that time. I'm so glad we did that. It would have been so easy to drown our sorrows. I'm not judging anybody—everyone's different and maybe it's fine for some people—but for us, I think not drinking during that most intense period was really a good thing.

David McGinnis

If you see something is going on with a family member, and it's about something sensitive, like alcohol or drugs or PTSD symptoms, approach the question gradually. Pretend you don't know anything—don't analyze or diagnose—just ask questions. Maybe start talking about something you read in the newspaper, like "I read a story today about a lot of veterans who are feeling depressed after they come home." Start general, then bring it around to the specific, like: "Have you ever felt like that?" You don't want to put them on the defensive, if you can help it.

5. Your Mission: Improve Function

This chapter will answer the following questions:

What's the goal in treating acute pain?

Why is the goal different for treating versus managing chronic pain?

What does "improving function" mean in the real world?

If you can't measure pain, how can you tell if a treatment is working?

How can you measure progress toward functional goals?

Which healthcare professionals, aside from your doctor, are you likely to be working with in order to accomplish the mission of reducing pain and improving function?

Looking beyond Pain Relief

The military trained me to look at life situations in terms of missions. I think that's a good way to go for pain relief, too. If you can define your mission clearly, and the steps you need to take to accomplish it, you have a much

greater chance of succeeding. The trick is to make sure
you're choosing the *right* mission. When it comes to pain,
especially chronic pain, you need to be careful. If you
break a bone, have a toothache, or burn yourself, you're
feeling acute pain and you want it to stop. Fair enough.
Both you and your doctor (if you need one) will focus on
eliminating the pain and fixing whatever is wrong. The
mission goal for acute pain, therefore, is straightforward:
pain relief. Determining if you're making progress in the
mission is pretty simple, too: If you're still feeling pain,
the mission is failing.

It's a different story with chronic pain. Although it
might sound odd, the mission goal for treating chronic
pain is not *only* pain relief. If you make pain relief your
sole focus, you're going to miss your target. It's very easy
to get tripped up in this way. You can succeed completely
in dulling or even eliminating your pain yet fail at everything else in your life. That's what I want to talk about in
this chapter: the idea that your mission is more than reducing your pain. It's about restoring function and regaining
your quality of life.

For me, the mission was all about regaining lost function. Controlling my pain was not the end—*it was the
means to the end*. I wanted to walk again. I wanted to run.
I wanted to drive. I wanted to surf, and ride my bike, and
have as close to an ordinary life as I could. I needed to find
ways to decrease my pain with the right use of medications
without compromising my focus or becoming sedated or
fuzzy. I didn't want to become so obsessed with getting
pain relief that I took my eyes off my larger goals, and in
the process, slowly lost function.

Because chronic pain is, by definition, a long-term
problem, it is extremely likely that by the time those with

VOICES OF SURVIVAL

Melissa Stockwell was commissioned as an officer in the U.S. Army in May 2002, after which she received training as a transportation officer. She was deployed to Iraq in March 2004 and quickly found out that a transportation officer's job is as dangerous as any other soldier's.

Melissa was in the lead vehicle of a convoy heading toward Baghdad when it was hit by an IED. Her vehicle slammed into a guardrail and crashed into a house. Between the blast and the crash, Melissa lost her left leg above the knee.

She woke up in a Baghdad military hospital. Her husband, Dave, also serving in Iraq, was there. She says they made an immediate decision: "Let's get on with this, and on with life."

From Iraq, Melissa was flown to Landstuhl and then to Walter Reed, where she spent a year in recovery and rehabilitation. She underwent 15 surgeries in all and says the treatment she received at Walter Reed was the "best care in the world," adding, "the rehab was wonderful."

Melissa is now fully mobile. She has even relearned to ski. "Skiing was absolutely the best experience I had after being hurt. I felt so free just to fly down the side of a mountain."

She is now earning a bachelor's degree in prosthetics from Century College in Minnesota. She says she felt "absolute joy" when she made a prosthetic leg for a 10-year-old girl, and watched the child put the leg on then get up and jump around. In the future, she is hoping to help wounded service members coming back from Iraq and Afghanistan get their lives back through prosthetic care.

chronic pain seek help they will be living in a state of reduced functioning. They may not be sleeping well, they
may not be exercising, or enjoying recreational activities,
or being intimate, or working to their full potential at their
jobs. This is what I mean by "functioning." The ultimate
goal of chronic pain treatment—the real mission—is to restore you to a healthy level of functioning.

Here are some of the main benefits of framing your
mission in terms of improving function:

> ❂ Both you and your doctor have objective, verifiable
> treatment goals and outcomes, as opposed to untestable
> and subjective ones such as simply "feeling better."

> ❂ Individual differences among patients, in terms of
> pain tolerance and functional goals, are easily accom-
> modated.

> ❂ A set of functional goals provides a solid basis for
> making decisions about whether or not to increase or
> decrease dosages, or switch to other forms of medica-
> tion altogether.

> ❂ A function-based treatment strategy is much more
> likely to improve your overall quality of life.

It's important to remember that dealing with chronic pain is a long-term mission—a marathon, not a sprint.
Your goals in the beginning might be incredibly modest.
For example, my first functional milepost toward my ultimate goal of running again was to be able to stand up and
balance using my prosthetic. Once I mastered that—and it
took practice—I could try taking one step. Once I mastered

walking on a level surface, I could try an incline. I freely admit that I wasn't always a good patient in this regard. I wanted to run *now*, and I sometimes pushed my body too hard and paid for it with increased pain or a lack of progress. Sometimes I still push too hard—though I think I'm getting smarter about training over time. My point is that setting functional goals is an ongoing process that evolves as your functioning improves. The more function you recover, the more ambitious your goals can become.

How Much Pain Relief Is Enough?

A critical part of a function-based mission is determining how much pain you are willing to tolerate. The traditional 0–to–10 pain scale used so often in clinics and hospitals inadvertently implies that the ideal condition is zero pain. In truth, hardly anybody lives with zero pain. I certainly don't! Even perfectly healthy, uninjured people feel low-grade pain of various kinds—aches, itches, or cramps, for example. It's a matter of how you cope with it and how you find the treatments and the methods that allow you to live a happy, functioning life.

For patients in chronic pain, the goal, therefore, is not zero pain, but acceptable pain. What's acceptable for one person may not be for another. We all have different levels of pain tolerance. The key is to find the level of pain that you can live with and that allows you to function at work and home, as well as to pursue personal passions.

Most people in chronic pain certainly need to feel some reduction in their pain, but it may not need to be as much as they think, if at the same time they are making obvious progress toward their functional goals. You often need to take an experimental approach to finding the best trade-off between pain relief and gaining (or keeping) the level of functioning you want, especially if the pain relief involves opioid medications. The dose of medication (or the use of other treatments) must be balanced with the amount of function they allow. You should use a medication or treatment as long as it is helping you reach your functional goals and overall mission. If the treatment begins to get in the way of those goals, you should seek out other treatments.

Building a Team

Successfully treating chronic pain usually requires that you assemble a team of professionals who can help you achieve your functional goals. If you are fortunate, one member of the team will be a pain specialist. Pain specialists are usually healthcare providers who have additional training in pain medicine and/or board certification in pain medicine. They look for a balance of different treatments tailored to each person's needs. Unfortunately, there are not yet enough pain specialists in either the military or civilian healthcare systems; but it is worth pursuing because pain medicine is a large, complex medical specialty, and most primary care physicians don't have the time to keep abreast of the rapid changes in this field.

Because many OIF/OEF veterans like myself sustain complex wounds that involve many body systems, many different specialists may be required for comprehensive care. They may include:

- Physical therapists (PTs)
- Occupational therapists

- ✪ Neurologists
- ✪ Speech therapists
- ✪ Vision therapists
- ✪ Psychiatrists
- ✪ Psychologists or counselors
- ✪ Social workers
- ✪ Prosthetists
- ✪ Complementary and alternative medicine practitioners
- ✪ Physiatrists (specialists in physical medicine and rehabilitation)

I saw all of these specialists at one time or another, and continue to use their services when I need them.

When you're working with healthcare professionals of any kind, the first step is to take an active role—don't be passive. A lot of people, whether they realize it or not, think that it's the doctor's job to fix whatever is broken in their body or mind. They don't realize that, in fact, the doctor isn't really in charge of their recovery. Your role is more like commanding officer of a battalion. Your doctor and the other specialists are like military specialists in communication, artillery, logistics, and navigation. They have expertise you must rely upon, and can offer advice you need. But, at the end of the day, you're the one who calls the shots; you are, ultimately, the one responsible for the success or failure of your mission. I will always be deeply thankful for all of the doctors, nurses and, other professionals who saved

> The good physician treats the disease; the great physician treats the patient who has the disease.
> —William Osler, physician 1849–1919

my life, repaired my eyes, stitched my wounds, retrained my brain, and gave me the tools I needed to recover. But none of those excellent people was ultimately responsible for me being able to walk again, or run, or do any of the other things I can now do. In fact, from my point of view, they had the easy part—fixing the bones and tissues. The hard part was living through all of the ups and downs of recovery and of working for months and months to slowly recover the functions I had lost. That's just the nature of recovery—and if I can do it, you can too.

Now that you have a strategic overview of your pain management mission, you're ready to learn about the arsenal of treatment options that you and your healthcare team can use to accomplish it, and that's the subject of the next chapter.

THE FAMILY JOURNEY

There are many ways family members can work with an injured service member to help him or her achieve the kinds of functional goals I have talked about in this chapter. In fact, family members are the ones on the front lines here, not the doctors, nurses, and other healthcare professionals. For one thing, family members know what a service member was like before he or she was injured. That knowledge can serve as a baseline or benchmark against which to set goals and assess progress. In addition, many functional goals involve factors that family members are ideally positioned to observe: sleep habits, exercise levels, mood, energy, ability to participate socially, and more. There are also a number of functional goals that are impossible to achieve without the participation of certain family members. Resumption of sexual activity is an obvious example; but others, such as resuming social activities that involve partners (e.g., dancing, playing bridge, bowling) can be equally important. Here are some other ways you can help a loved one make steady progress toward his or her functional goals:

✪ If possible, go with your family member to meetings with doctors and other caregivers.

✪ If a functional goal is not being pursued, or a functional approach to pain management is not being taken, look for a doctor or pain specialist who will use this approach. (Visit the Exit Wounds website for links to resources to help you locate healthcare providers in your area.)

✪ Once a set of goals has been established, provide support in the form of gentle reminders, encouragement, and words of praise. No need to nag—let your family member know that you care and want to help him or her succeed any way you can.

✪ Encourage patience. Achieving functional goals, especially if it involves the healing of major wounds, is a slow process. Remember: it's a marathon, not a sprint.

✪ Agree that you be allowed to call the doctor directly if you feel there is a problem or if you see that your family member is not reaching his or her functional goals.

Having this agreement in place early is key; if you wait until later, a service member may feel you are overstepping your role. Make it clear that this is a team effort and that you are a vital part of the "command and control" structure!

Andrea

If you think your partner is stuck in their efforts to reach a goal, or if you can't seem to help them get motivated to keep trying, find somebody in your partner's care circle—a friend, doctor, case manager, relatives—somebody you think they'll listen to. Explain things to them and have them talk to your partner.

David McGinnis

Family members can help by trying to keep the big picture in mind. Your family member can get so focused on stopping the pain that it can help to just gently remind them of their long-term goals, whatever those might be.

6. Your Arsenal of Treatment Options

This chapter will answer the following questions:

What are the different categories of pain relievers?

What are opioids and how can they best be used to manage chronic pain?

What's the difference between tolerance and addiction?

Are there other types of medications besides opioids that are used to help fight pain?

Which rehabilitation techniques can help with chronic pain?

What are injection and infusion therapies?

What are implantable devices and when are they appropriate?

Which surgical interventions can help reduce chronic pain?

How can you best use complementary and alternative medicine techniques?

What are the latest treatments for phantom limb pain?

Treating the Whole Person

In the course of my recovery from the injuries I sustained from the IED in Iraq, I used nearly every form of possible pain treatment, from acupuncture to nerve blocks and practically everything in between. I'm not saying that makes me a pain specialist; I'm not, which is why I developed the material in this chapter based on the APF's *Treatment Options: A Guide to People Living with Pain,* and with the help of the folks I mentioned in the introduction—real experts in pain management. What I do have is extensive personal experience with most of these techniques, which has taught me a lot about some general principles of pain management.

To begin with, it's important to keep in mind as you read here that pain is complex and highly individual. Just because a given technique worked for me doesn't mean it will work for you. To give you an example: the doctors at Walter Reed called in an acupuncturist in an attempt to relieve the extreme pain I was feeling in my injured leg. It didn't work for me, because, as we later learned, the problem was not something acupuncture could realistically address. Still, it was a valiant attempt, and I give the doctors credit for trying it; but the solution in my case had nothing to do with trying to dull the pain and everything to do with surgically eliminating the cause of that pain—the bone spurs and abnormal bursa at the tip of the severed femur. Once those were corrected, everything began to improve and my pain eased tremendously.

I've said it before, but it bears repeating, there is no one-size-fits-all treatment for pain. Not only do people differ in their basic anatomy and physiology, they also have unique pain responses based on differences in their upbringing, beliefs about pain, and general cultural environment. These differences mean that you need to work with your doctor (and pain management team, if you have one) to map out a treatment plan tailored to your specific needs. The overall goal is to improve your functioning and enhance your quality of life. Lowering your pain level is one step toward accomplishing those missions.

Another lesson I've learned, and seen demonstrated by my fellow veterans, is that in many cases a combination of treatments works better than just one treatment. This is called a "multimodality" approach. For example, your healthcare provider may prescribe a medication, along with activities to reduce stress, such as yoga or physical therapy. As I've described, chronic pain can affect every sphere of life, meaning you may need to treat several issues at the same time, such as the pain itself plus anxiety and sleep difficulties. The idea is to treat the entire person, not just one body part or one area of functioning. That's what "holistic" or "integrative" treatment means—and it's the best way to approach your overall treatment and recovery.

Finally, I think it's helpful to frame the big picture of treating pain as a balance of risks and benefits. All treatments—even plain old aspirin—carry some degree of risk. Some medications or treatments carry higher degrees of risk, which means they are most appropriate when the benefits they deliver outweigh those risks. This risk/benefit equation usually changes as your treatment progresses. A treatment that was worth using initially, despite some risks, may no longer be appropriate if your level of pain has been brought under control. The key point: constantly evaluate, and reevaluate, your pain and whatever treatment you might be using to make sure you continue to reap maximum benefits with the lowest risk.

In this chapter I'll review the most common treatment options in seven broad categories:

- ✪ Medications
- ✪ Psychosocial treatments
- ✪ Physical rehabilitation
- ✪ Injection and infusion devices
- ✪ Implantable devices
- ✪ Treatments for phantom limb pain
- ✪ Complementary and alternative techniques

I'll be giving you just an overview here so that you understand the range of potential treatments and how they can fit together as part of a holistic treatment plan. Be aware there's a great deal to learn about each option, and when it comes to pain management, information is power. The more you know about your pain condition, the more effectively you can collaborate with your medical team.

For more detailed and updated information, resources, and links, go to the Exit Wounds website. Pain medicine is a fast-moving field, and new developments are emerging all the time, so it's a good idea to stay current.

Keeping a Pain Diary

Regardless of the type of treatment, or treatments, you pursue, it can be extremely helpful for yourself and your care team to keep a pain diary or notebook. For more about this, check out the American Pain Foundation's publication, "Target Chronic Pain Notebook." You can print out this notebook to use at home; it's available for download from www.painfoundation.org and the Exit Wounds website. In it you can record your pain experience (when it occurs, for how long, the level and type of pain, possible triggers, etc.), its impact on your day-to-day life (which activities you can or cannot do), and how you respond to various treatments over time, including side effects and improvements in daily function and emotional wellness.

Finding the right combination of treatments to relieve pain may take time and patience. By keeping track of what makes your pain better or worse, you will help your healthcare team find the best treatment approach for you. Plus you'll be playing a more active role in your care, which can help you stay positive and feel more in control.

Medications

Anti-inflammatories

Aspirin, which was introduced as a pain reliever in 1899, is the founding member of a class of medications now called nonsteroidal anti-inflammatory drugs, or NSAIDs. All NSAIDs relieve mild to moderate pain and reduce fever and inflammation. They work by decreasing the formation of natural substances in the body called prostaglandins, which are produced at sites of injury or swelling and make nearby pain receptors more sensitive. By slowing the release of prostaglandins, NSAIDs reduce pain and inflammation. But prostaglandins also help protect a number of areas in the body such as the stomach and kidneys, so NSAIDs, which reach the entire body, may cause side effects such as stomach upset or kidney problems.

Aspirin, ibuprofen, naproxen sodium, and ketoprofen are the only classes of NSAIDs available without a prescription. A different class of NSAIDs, selective COX–2 inhibitors, were developed to reduce the risk of ulcers caused by NSAIDs. Only one selective COX-2 inhibitor, celecoxib, is still available at this time, and it is available by prescription only.

In addition to treating mild to moderate pain, NSAIDs are important for the management of both acute and chronic pain. They are the go-to treatment for run-of-the-mill acute pain from minor injuries. NSAIDS are also commonly used in combination with other drugs such as opioids for treating more severe pain. But NSAIDs alone are not effective treatments for chronic pain.

There is no evidence that one NSAID is a better pain reliever than another; however, each individual may get better pain relief from one than from another. That means finding the right NSAID to treat persistent pain is a matter of trial and error. Also, note that it might take awhile for the drug to work, so you and your provider will need to allow for an adequate time trial of the drug before judging its benefit.

NSAIDs have an important limitation, called a "dose ceiling." Taking doses above the ceiling will significantly raise the risk of serious side effects, such as kidney failure, which can be life-threatening.

Common side effects of NSAIDs include:

- Stomach upset
- Stomach ulcers
- Gastrointestinal (GI) bleeding
- Delayed blood clotting
- Decreased kidney function
- Possible higher risk of stroke or heart attack with selective COX–2 inhibitors

Acetaminophen

Like an NSAID, acetaminophen can relieve mild to moderate pain and treat fever; but it is *not* an NSAID and will not reduce swelling. It produces few, if any, side effects at the doses that can relieve pain, but it can damage the liver when used in large doses, especially if used with alcohol. The labeling specifies an upper limit of 4000 mg/24 hours (the equivalent to eight extra-strength tablets). If you have liver disease or a history of alcohol abuse, you should limit your use of acetaminophen and talk to your doctor about other types of pain relievers.

As with NSAIDs, acetaminophen is often combined with an opioid medication—usually, in the same pill or capsule—to treat moderate to severe pain. Be sure to check the amount with your doctor or pharmacist. Don't decide on your own to take extra acetaminophen if a combination pain medicine is not controlling your pain, because you could end up using too much acetaminophen, and that could cause liver damage. Currently, there is concern in the medical community about the growing rate of liver damage associated with large doses of acetaminophen. Make sure to speak to your healthcare provider to monitor the amount of acetaminophen you are taking. You should also be aware that many over-the-counter (OTC) cough, cold, and sinus remedies contain acetaminophen.

Possible side effects of acetaminophen include:

- Possible liver damage at high doses
- Liver damage and stomach bleeding if used in combination with alcohol

Opioids

Many veterans of Operation Enduring Freedom have probably seen the flowers of the opium poppy, because some 500,000 acres of this plant are under cultivation in Afghanistan. The principal active drug in opium is morphine. Morphine was the first in what is now a very large class of pain relievers called **opioids**. Many of these drugs are made synthetically today, although some drug companies continue to grow and harvest vast expanses of opium poppies to acquire the raw materials for modern pain medications.

Opioids: Medications that mimic the pain-reducing effects of opium in the body. Some opioid drugs are made from extracts of opium poppies. Others are synthetic drugs made to behave in similar ways to opium.

The pain-relieving properties of opioids are unsurpassed; they are today considered the "gold standard" of pain medications, and so are often the main medications used in the treatment of chronic pain. Yet, despite their great benefits, opioids are often underused. For a number of reasons, healthcare providers may be afraid to prescribe them, and patients may be afraid to take them. At the core of this wariness is the fear of addiction, so I want to tackle this issue head-on.

If your body adjusts to a drug or medication, it may become less effective over time. This is called **tolerance**. This is simply a physiological process that doesn't occur for all people or with all medications. Many people with persistent pain, for example, *don't* develop tolerance and stay on the same dose of opioids for a long time. **Physical dependence** means that a person will develop symptoms and signs of withdrawal (e.g., sweating, rapid heart rate, nausea, diarrhea, goose bumps, or anxiety) if a drug or medication is suddenly stopped or the dose is lowered too quickly. Withdrawal can be a problem with many medications used on a long-term basis, such as antidepressants, anticonvulsants, and medicines prescribed to control high blood pressure. Physical dependence is normal. This does not mean you are addicted.

Opioid medications can, however, be abused or used as recreational drugs, and some people who use these drugs this way *will* become addicted. **Addiction** is a disease state in which people can no longer control their use of a drug that is causing them harm. They continue to crave and use the drug despite the harm it may be causing to their health, their relationships, or their ability to function in other spheres of life. Smoking cigarettes is the most common form of addiction in the United States today; alcohol addiction is the next most common.

Long experience with opioids shows that people who are not predisposed to addiction are unlikely to become addicted to opioid pain medications. When used correctly, opioid pain medications *increase* a person's level of functioning; conversely, when a drug is used by somebody who is addicted, his or her function *decreases.*

Doctors will typically ask patients if they or any

Tolerance: The adaptation of the body to the presence of a medication such that higher doses are required to receive the same therapeutic benefit as the original dose.

Physical dependence: A nondisease state common to patients taking a wide variety of medications. It means the patient's body has adjusted to a medication and that if the medication is stopped suddenly, withdrawal symptoms will set in.

Addiction: A disease state in which a person can no longer control his or her use of a drug that is causing harm. Using the drug decreases functioning at work, at home, and in relationships, and causes health problems.

close relatives have a history of addiction. Answering yes does not automatically disqualify a person from getting a prescription for opioids; it means only that both the patient and the physician will need to pay close attention to the use of the medication and watch for signs of addictive behaviors. The doctor may also ask the patient to sign a written treatment plan that spells out exactly how the medication will be prescribed and how future decisions to continue or end its use will be made. Denying a person opioid pain medication because he or she has a history of substance abuse or addiction is contrary to the model guidelines for prescribing opioids, published by the U.S. Federation of State Medical Boards.

Another reason opioid medications may not be used as often as perhaps they might be among service members is fear that such use might jeopardize their jobs. Say you've been trained as a fighter pilot, and you think you will be disqualified for that job if you have been prescribed an opioid medication. You may decide to "tough it out" so you can keep doing your job. I've seen this happen many times—in fact, I've felt this very same impulse myself. I can't offer a good solution to the problem, but I do think it deserves some careful attention from the military because the end result is likely to be service members who suffer needlessly; it also greatly increases the chance that they will, sooner or later, develop chronic pain.

Types of Opioids There are many classes of opioid pain medications. Some are fast-acting, some are long-lasting; some are more apt to make you sleepy; some are more or less likely to cause stomach upset. Fortunately, the range of medications and the many ways they can be delivered give your doctor numerous options to consider when prescribing the medication that will work best for you and your specific pain. This might require some experimentation, but the number of available medications makes it more likely you'll find one that works.

Here's a list of the more common types of opioids:

- Codeine
- Morphine
- Methadone
- Hydrocodone
- Oxycodone
- Hydromorphone
- Propoxyphene
- Fentanyl

As I said earlier, an opioid may be combined with acetaminophen or an NSAID. Combination medications have relatively low dose limitations because of the dangers of liver toxicity from the acetaminophen. For severe pain, pure opioids are used because their doses can be gradually increased over time if the pain intensifies.

One of the advantages of opioid medications is that they can be given in so many different ways: by mouth; as a rectal suppository; via intravenous injection (IV); subcutaneously (under the skin); transdermally (through the skin, via a patch) or into a region around the spinal cord. Patches, IV injections, and infusions are very important for patients who cannot swallow or whose GI tracts are not working normally.

Opioids also vary in their duration of effect. "Ordinary" opioid medications (i.e., ones not altered to extend their effects) only provide several hours of pain relief after a dose. Short-acting opioids may be prescribed for breakthrough pain, severe flares of pain that may "break through" a stable and comfortable state for short periods of time. Extended-release formulations can provide pain relief from 8 to 24 hours; and some medications can be delivered via a patch that can provide relief for as long as 72 hours.

Side Effects of Opioids Finding the medication, dose, and delivery route that works best for you is often a matter of balancing the benefits of the medication against the side effects it produces. You and your doctor will seek the most benefit with the least side effects—which, again, is highly individual.

The most common side effects of opioids are:

- ✪ Constipation
- ✪ Nausea and vomiting
- ✪ Sleepiness
- ✪ Mental cloudiness
- ✪ Itching
- ✪ Dizziness
- ✪ Difficulty urinating

The good news is that, with the exception of constipation, most side effects disappear after a few days for most (not all) people. In regard to constipation, some pain experts believe all patients started on an opioid also should be taking a stool softener or a laxative. Others believe that this treatment is appropriate only if a patient is prone to developing serious constipation, because of advanced age, poor diet, other diseases, or the use of other constipating drugs. Your healthcare provider can give you advice on diet and which medicines to use to treat constipation. If you experience any other side effects that don't go away in the expected time frame, tell your doctor. Perhaps you can try another type of opioid, or there may be ways to treat the side effects with another medication.

The bottom line with opioids is that these are very valuable pain relievers *when used correctly and responsibly*, and they can go a long way toward improving your functioning in daily life. The keys, as always, are to have good communication with your healthcare provider, be persistent, and keep a positive attitude.

Medications for Neuropathic Pain

Neuropathic pain is caused by damaged nerves, rather than by actual injury or tissue damage. For a variety of reasons, this makes neuropathic pain more difficult to treat than acute pain. (I discuss phantom limb pain, a special case of neuropathic pain, later in this chapter.) Drugs from several different classes, including certain antidepressants, anticonvulsants, and corticosteroids, have been found to help relieve neuropathic pain. Certain opioids, too, may be used. Often, a combination of drugs will provide the best relief; for example, a recent study confirmed that combining gabapentin and morphine gives better relief for neuropathic pain than using either one alone.

A partial list of the medications commonly used for neuropathic pain:

- Opioid analgesics and tramadol
- Lidocaine patch
- Antidepressants, in particular, tricyclic medications, venlafaxine, and duloxetine
- Anticonvulsants, such as gabapentin and pregabalin
- Corticosteroids, if pain is due to inflammation

Each of these agents may produce a different array of side effects, which your doctor should review with you prior to prescribing.

To learn more about the side effects of pain medications, visit the Exit Wounds website.

Physical Rehabilitation

Physical methods have been used for centuries to relieve pain. Today, numerous types of healthcare professionals with specialized training use physical techniques to help reduce pain. Many work in the field of rehabilitative medicine, including physiatrists (physicians who specialize in physical medicine), physical therapists, occupational therapists, and exercise physiologists. Some forms of physical rehabilitation involve hands-on manipulations such as deep-tissue massage, while others use devices such as transcutaneous electrical stimulation.

Physiatry

Physiatrists provide a wide variety of treatments for the musculoskeletal system (the muscles and bones); they do not perform surgery. Because the back is the core of the musculoskeletal system, many physiatrists are considered specialists in treating back pain. A number of physiatrists have additional training in special areas, like sports medicine, brain or spinal cord injury, or pain management.

Physical Therapy

Physical therapists (PTs) help restore function, improve mobility, and relieve pain. If you have suffered a serious wound during service, it is very likely that you'll work with a PT in the course of your recovery. You'll first be tested to assess your strength, range of motion, balance and coordination, posture, muscle performance, respiration, and motor function. Then an individualized plan will be drawn up to maximize your independence and function.

Physical therapists use a variety of treatment methods to relieve pain and reduce swelling, including electrical stimulation, hot packs, cold compresses, traction, deep tissue massage, and ultrasound. They also teach patients to use assistive or adaptive devices, such as crutches, prostheses, and wheelchairs. Exercise training is often provided, which can be performed at home to help advance recovery by reducing increasing mobility and improving flexibility, strength, and/or endurance. As treatment continues, physical therapists will document your progress, conduct periodic examinations, and modify therapies, as necessary.

Occupational Therapy

Occupational therapists (OTs) will help you learn to perform tasks required for daily living and in the work setting. These include a wide range of activities, from using a computer to mastering everyday basics such as dressing, cooking, and eating. Physical exercises may be used to increase strength and skillfulness. Occupational therapists also instruct those with disabilities in the use of adaptive equipment, including wheelchairs, splints, and aids for eating and dressing. They can design or make special equipment needed at home or at work.

Hydrotherapy

Hydrotherapy is the use of water to aid in health maintenance or to promote healing. Also known as aquatic or pool therapy, the use of therapeutically warm water and exercise may help ease the pain in muscles and joints. Gentle movement in the water may help build strength and relax stiff joints and sore muscles; and water buoyancy greatly reduces the pressure on joints, making it easier to perform range-of-motion exercises. Hydrotherapy is now a part of the physical therapy department of virtually every hospital and medical center. I found hydrotherapy to be very effective in helping to relieve some of my phantom limb pain and sensations.

Transcutaneous Electrical Nerve Stimulation (TENS)

TENS is a method of physical therapy that attempts to decrease pain without needles or surgery. The TENS unit is designed to block or prevent pain by providing opposing stimulation to compete with the unpleasant signals that cause pain. TENS can be used in the treatment of acute and chronic pain, including pain of the lower back, neck, pelvis, nerves, and muscles.

Used properly, TENS units are very safe, and do not hurt. The best time to wear a TENS unit is during activities or times of the day when your pain is generally the most severe. The sensation should feel comfortable or pleasurable when the unit is turned on. The units are battery-operated (9–volt), hence should *not* be worn in the shower or bathtub.

Complementary and Alternative Medicine

Complementary and alternative techniques encompass many medical and healthcare systems, practices, and products that are not presently considered part of conventional medicine. They are, however, best used in combination with medications or more conventional approaches, an approach known as **integrative medicine**. Some of these techniques, such as acupuncture, are widely used and accepted by the medical community; others, such as homeopathy, are not currently in widespread use, although some people claim benefits from them. Here, I'll focus on techniques known to be helpful for alleviating pain.

> *Complementary medicine:* Therapies or techniques such as acupuncture that are used along with traditional (western) medical techniques.
> *Alternative medicine:* Therapies or techniques used *in place of* western medical practices.
> *Integrative medicine:* The combination of conventional medical therapies and complementary and alternative medicine therapies for which there is some high-quality scientific evidence of safety and effectiveness.

Acupuncture

Acupuncture has a growing acceptance in the field of western conventional medicine; in eastern cultures, it has been practiced for thousands of years. Today, acupuncture describes a family of procedures involving stimulation of anatomical points on the body by a variety of techniques. The American practice of acupuncture incorporates the ancient medical traditions of China, Japan, Korea, and other countries. The acupuncture technique that has been widely studied scientifically in this country involves penetrating the skin with thin metallic needles that are manipulated by the practitioner's hands or by electrical stimulation.

People experience acupuncture differently, but most feel no or minimal pain as the needles are inserted and in place. Some people feel energized following treatment, while others feel relaxed. Improper needle placement, movement of the patient while the needles are in place, or a defect in a needle can cause soreness and pain during or after treatment. This is why it is important to seek treatment from a qualified acupuncture practitioner. (Note that most states require a license to practice acupuncture, and the FDA regulates the manufacture and labeling of acupuncture needles.)

A related technique is acupressure, which is based on the same Chinese theories that underlie acupuncture. In acupressure, the practitioner uses his or her hands and/or fingers, rather than needles, to apply stimulation. Acupressure relaxes muscular tension and balances what are believed to be the vital life forces of the body. The patient lies fully clothed on a soft massage table while the practitioner presses gently on meridian points situated on various parts of the body. According to the theory behind acupuncture, these points are the pathways along which the body's vital energy flows. The session is noninvasive and gentle. An average session lasts for about one hour, and most people require a number of sessions to complete a treatment.

Chiropractic Care

The chiropractic therapeutic approach focuses on the relationship between bodily structure (primarily that of the spine) and function, and how this relationship affects the protection and restoration of health. Chiropractors use spinal manipulative therapy as a basic treatment tool. The primary principle of the chiropractic profession promotes a natural method of healthcare that includes respect for the human body's ability to heal itself, without the use of surgery or medication. Chiropractors give careful attention to the biomechanics, structure, and function of the spine; its effects on the musculoskeletal and neurological systems; and the role played by the proper function of these systems in the preservation and restoration of health.

Chiropractors frequently treat individuals with a variety of pain disorders, such as headaches, joint pain, neck pain, low back pain, and sciatica.

Massage

Massage therapists manipulate muscle and connective tissue to enhance function of those tissues and promote relaxation and well-being. Massage is an old healing art with many techniques and approaches. Massage acts directly on the nervous system to promote relaxation. It can ease painful, tight muscles, and releases spasm by stretching and gently separating individual muscle fibers that may have become bound and knotted together.

Massage can help increase range of motion in joints, enhance blood circulation, and relieve pain. Massage may also promote a restful sleep by helping the body and mind relax.

Guided Imagery and Visualization

The connections between the mind and body mean that the mind can be harnessed to affect the body in beneficial ways. Guided imagery and visualization are forms of meditation in which one's thoughts are guided toward patterns and images that help relieve pain, promote healing from injury or illness, and/or ease depression, anxiety, and sleeplessness.

Imagery relaxes the body by aiding the release of brain chemicals that serve as the body's natural tranquilizers. These chemicals lower blood pressure, heart rate, and anxiety levels. Several studies suggest that imagery can also boost the immune system and, therefore, promote healing.

Most guided imagery techniques begin with relaxation followed by the visualization of a mental image. A leader might, for example, have patients imagine a color for pain and then have them gradually replace that color with one that is more pleasing. Another common technique is visualizing a peaceful scene, such as the ocean surf or a wooded forest. Learning to harness your mind to reduce stress and promote calm may provide you with a long-term tool to help reduce chronic pain.

Injection and Infusion Therapies

This class of pain treatment involves either an injection (one-time, rapid) or an infusion (slow delivery over a longer time period) of pain medications, or some other type of treatment such as electricity, heat, or cold. These methods may be used to prevent or control both acute and chronic pain.

Injection Therapies (Nerve Blocks)

Injection therapies may be used to treat painful conditions in many areas of the body. Also called "nerve blocks," these techniques involve placing a needle into a muscle, joint, spine, or around a specific group of nerves, followed by the injection of medication(s) or delivery of some other treatment such as electricity, heat, or cold.

Nerve blocks can be used to help determine whether your pain is coming from a specific nerve, muscle, or joint, and which one. Certain kinds of nerve blocks are first done with a local anesthetic medication. If you feel relief, a more permanent type of block may be recommended. Nerve blocks can also be used to prevent development of chronic pain syndromes (prophylactic nerve blocks). Therapeutic nerve blocks may reduce pain, either alone or as a complement to other pain treatment options.

Interestingly, the use of nerve blocks in acute care delivered on the battlefield is becoming more and more accepted. Because they are a form of local anesthetic, nerve blocks have some distinct advantages as part of trauma care over medications that affect the entire body. In addition, some studies suggest that by blocking the transmission of pain signals to the brain, you reduce the chance that pain may become "hardwired" into the body after the wound has healed, causing chronic or persistent pain. Research into this connection between the treatment of acute pain and the risk of later chronic pain is a very active field of study at the moment.

Neuroablative Therapies

Neuroablative therapies usually produce a longer-lasting effect than nerve blocks. These therapies use thermal (heat or cold) or chemical agents (alcohol or phenol) to destroy or incapacitate certain nerves, thereby providing prolonged pain relief. Your pain specialist might choose this option if your pain is severe, expected to persist, and cannot be eased by other therapies.

Infusion Therapies

Infusion therapies, especially intravenous (IV) drug delivery, can be an effective way to control your pain. Giving pain medications through a small tube, placed under the skin, in your vein, or in your spine, provides faster and more effective pain relief than medications taken by mouth. These methods are commonly used after surgery, injury, or trauma.

Delivery of a medication under the skin can be very helpful for people in chronic pain. A small needle is placed under your skin into your subcutaneous, or "fatty," tissue. The needle is connected to a tube and infusion pump, which delivers the pain medication into the tissue. Subcutaneous infusion can successfully be used at home after you are trained to do so.

Infusing pain medications and/or local anesthetics near or directly into the spinal fluid space within the spine (epidural analgesia) is sometimes used after surgery, painful injury, or illness. This can give you better pain relief and help you move more easily and quickly after surgery. It is also possible to use less pain medicine and have fewer side effects, which should speed your recovery.

Chronic neuropathic pain may be alleviated with infusions of a local anesthetic such as lidocaine. The local anesthetic is given over a 30- to 60-minute period of time and is usually done in an outpatient or ambulatory care setting.

Implantable Devices

Spinal Cord Stimulation

Spinal cord stimulation (SCS) involves the use of a small battery-powered device, called a pulse generator or receiver, to deliver electrical impulses to nerves along the spinal cord. These impulses interfere with the transmission of pain signals to the brain. When successful, you feel a mild tingling sensation instead of pain. SCS may be used to treat chronic neuropathic pain in the neck, arms, chest, back, or legs. Your doctor or pain specialist will perform an SCS trial to see if the therapy will help relieve your pain. If the trial is successful, an SCS system will be surgically implanted.

Implantable Pain Medication Pumps

Sometimes the best way to deliver a pain medicine is with a small surgically implanted pump. This is called intraspinal drug delivery and it allows for a continuous infusion of pain medications, possibly including opioids, local anesthetic drugs, or other drugs into your spinal fluid.

The implanted drug delivery system consists of a small flexible catheter placed in the spinal fluid and connected to a drug infusion pump, which is implanted under the skin of your abdomen. The medication is placed into the pump by a pain specialist or nurse, and the medication is slowly administered by the pump, which is programmed for how much of the drug you are to receive per day. As with any surgical procedure, your pain specialist or physician should provide you with detailed information on the therapy, system components, benefits and risks, and potential complications. This information can help you decide if intraspinal drug delivery is right for you.

See the Exit Wounds website for more detailed information on implantable treatment options and to download a free book from the American Pain Foundation about pain treatment options.

Treatments for Phantom Limb Pain

As of late 2008, nearly 900 U.S. service members have lost
at least one limb while serving in Iraq and Afghanistan,
according to the Pentagon. Most of these amputees, myself included, experience the sensation that the limb is still
there (called "phantom sensation"); and in the first year after loss of a limb, roughly 90 percent will experience phantom pain as well, which I described in Chapter 3. (The
percentage who continue to feel phantom pain drops slowly over time.) Because it is a type of neuropathic pain, and
because the pain can be complicated and exacerbated by
the fit and use of prostheses, phantom limb pain can be
difficult to treat. Nonetheless, you should be hopeful that
you will find relief and be able to use a prosthetic to regain
lost functioning. My own story is not unusual, both in the
amount of time and energy it took to finally achieve my
goals, and in the degree of freedom I now have to walk,
run, and engage in sports.

All of the techniques discussed above, particularly the
medications for neuropathic pain and some of the implanted electrical stimulator devices, are used to help manage
phantom limb pain. Again, because people vary tremendously in their responses to medications, and because the
condition of the remaining limbs also varies widely, it
will probably take some trial and error to find the best
medication(s), combined with a medical device or complementary therapy, to treat your phantom pain with a
minimum of side effects.

Two newly developed pain-relieving techniques are
specific to phantom pain and deserve attention. I'll review
them briefly here, and you can read more about them on
the Exit Wounds website.

VOICES OF SURVIVAL

On March 16, 2007, Army Sergeant Brandon Sword was part of a raid on a municipal building in the southern tip of the Sunni Triangle—an area known as the "triangle of death" because of its high casualty rate for U.S. troops. The team entered the building uneventfully and climbed to the roof. That's when a bomb embedded in the concrete was triggered.

"I saw a flash, an explosion, first," Brandon recalls. "It knocked me off my feet."

He fell to the ground, blood pouring from his head. He could move only his right arm and neck. He instructed one soldier to fasten a tourniquet on his left arm and left leg, and to bandage his head. The explosion destroyed the radio that had been wired to his helmet, so another soldier called for a Medevac chopper.

Brandon was treated for five days in Iraq then flown to Landstuhl for surgery to repair his many shrapnel wounds and apply skin grafts to large wounds on his legs. En route to the states, an artery ruptured in his head, forcing the plane to turn around. He finally made it home by the end of March and began a slow recovery that lasted through October of that year and involved 15 surgeries in all.

Although his wounds are now healed, Brandon has continued to suffer pain. "Your body is so riddled with injuries, your nerves get crossed, and they send these flashes to your brain," he explains.

Despite the pain, Brandon has forged ahead with his life. He was married in May 2007, and almost a year to the day after he was injured, his son Christian was born.

(*continued*)

(*Voices of Survival continued*)
Brandon and his wife, Stacy, now live in Wasilla, Alaska,
35 miles north of Anchorage, where they plan to start a
real estate investment company.

Brandon takes opioid medications, which give him
several hours of relief every day, and he is scheduled to
have a neurostimulator implanted soon.

"The stimulator is kind of like a new beginning,"
he says. "I want to have a lot more good days than I
do bad."

Mirror Box Therapy

This innovative treatment fights one illusion (phantom
pain) with another illusion: that the limb is no longer missing. Many amputees, myself among them, experience pain
as a clenched phantom limb in spasm or clenched digits
on a limb. The theory behind mirror box treatment is that
the brain interprets that a phantom limb is paralyzed because it has been receiving no feedback from the limb to in-
form it otherwise. Doctors at Walter Reed Army Medical
Center constructed a box that uses mirrors to reflect visu-
al feedback of a restored limb, which is passed on to the
brain.

Here's how it works: The intact limb is placed on one
side of the mirror, and in the patient's sight, while the re-
sidual limb is placed on the other side, out of sight. The
patient sees an intact second limb through the mirror and
tries to move both limbs at the same time. This effort, in
conjunction with the illusion of movement created by the
mirrors, gives the brain input that the phantom limb has
moved, too, and it becomes unparalyzed, thus relieving the

pain. Treatment with mirror box therapy can involve several weeks of therapy, once or twice a day.

Recent studies have found that mirror box therapy can reduce or eliminate phantom pain in most veterans who use it. In one study, 100 percent of those who used the therapy for four weeks reported a marked decrease in their pain, as measured on two types of pain scales. Consequently, this technique is being actively pursued by doctors in many medical hospitals. A good source of information about mirror therapy is the website of the Amputee Coalition of America (www.amputee-coalition.org) or the Exit Wounds website.

Deep Brain Stimulation

Deep brain stimulation is a surgical technique that has been shown to reduce or eliminate phantom pain in some patients. Using this technique, a neurosurgeon identifies nerves or regions of the brain that are active during a phantom pain experience. An electrode is then implanted in the identified area and connected to a pulse generator implanted under the skin of the upper chest. As with a spinal cord stimulator, the pulses generated by the electrode block or interfere with pain signals arriving at the brain.

Only a few studies of this technique have been done to date, but initial results are encouraging. In one study of three amputees, overall phantom pain was reduced by half, and the burning component of the pain was eliminated. Two of the amputees were able to cut back on their use of opioid medications, and all three reported significant improvements in their quality of life.

Planning for Relapse

Let's assume for the moment that you have used one or more of the treatments I've reviewed in this chapter, that your pain has been brought under control, and that you have regained lost functions. Now's the time that your healthcare team or pain specialist should talk to you about what to do if the pain comes back. Don't look at this as defeatist or pessimistic; it's a realistic and wise approach to dealing with a wily enemy. Remember, pain is a moving target. Your pain level can be affected by many things that change in life: the amount and nature of physical activity, stress, mood, or accidents involving a sensitive spot. Sometimes an existing condition, such as arthritis, will worsen, increasing pain levels; or nerves that had been "quiet" may for unknown reasons become resensitized.

Planning ahead for a recurrence of pain makes good sense, and it can give you the peace of mind that comes with being prepared. Planning may mean having a supply of a pain medication on hand, or the right types of heating and cooling pads to provide thermal treatments. The specifics of your "bad pain day" plan will be unique to you, your pain, and the nature of the wounds you have suffered.

Here are some other guidelines to keep in mind if you suffer a recurrence of pain:

✪ Remind yourself that you can manage your pain, rather than it managing you.

✪ Reach out for the support of others who can help with physical tasks or provide moral support.

✪ When asking for help, be as specific as possible in describing what you are experiencing.

✪ If pain persists for more than a day, or doesn't seem to respond to treatment, seek medical help—sooner rather than later.

✪ Get outside, if possible. Sometimes it can make all the difference in the world to take a walk, get some fresh air, and get your blood moving.

✪ Don't give in to despair. A recurrence does not mean a return to the frustrating days of prior suffering. If your pain was successfully treated at one point, it can be successfully treated again.

A Final Word

I hope you now see that your arsenal of potential pain treatments is formidable and ranges from learning breathing and relaxation techniques to the latest surgical and pharmacological treatments. At the same time, you need to know that not all of these options are available everywhere, and that not all physicians are familiar with these treatments, much less are experts in their use. What's important is that now you're aware they exist. Remember, the more you know about specific pain therapies, the more effectively you can advocate for treatment. To give yourself more ammunition, spend some time on the Exit Wounds website and explore the links to other authoritative sites you'll find there.

Never forget: If a treatment isn't working, there may be other options. You may need to push—hard—to get the attention and care you deserve from individual caregivers and/or from the often bureaucratic institutions in which they work. Keep at it! Everyone deserves full and effective pain treatment, but no one more so than those who have willingly put themselves in harm's way on behalf of their country!

THE FAMILY JOURNEY

Choosing which treatments to use for managing chronic pain is, of course, the decision of the person in pain, in cooperation with his or her team of caregivers. Still, family members can support pain treatment in many ways:

✪ Remind a service member to take medications according to the prescribed schedule. (This can be particularly important if the person is using opioid medications, as these can cause mental cloudiness, forgetfulness, and a failure to pay attention to time.)

✪ Encourage service members to consider nontraditional options for easing pain and raising comfort levels.

✪ Remain alert for signs of depression, anxiety, or post-combat stress reactions, as these can make pain worse and erode motivation to "stick with the program."

✪ Help with scheduling and making appointments with healthcare providers.

✪ Keep track of how much medication is left and make sure refills are ordered and obtained before they run out.

✪ Remind service members to keep prescription medications in a safe, secure location, out of the reach of children, and emphasize never to share their medications with others.

✪ Help service members create and maintain a medication schedule. If a brain injury is involved, this is a critical area of assistance.

Andrea

It's really important to take care of your own needs at the same time your partner is getting treatment or is in recovery. Do something for yourself, because your partner is going to be totally occupied with recovery or rehab. For me, it was always going to the gym to work out—that helped so much. But it could be anything—whatever you enjoy and helps you to relax.

These men and women who are injured are usually very well taken care of. Not just medically, but they get to go on trips, and have basketball teams come to visit them, and stuff like that. They get a lot of attention, and sometimes spouses sort of get left behind, and they get to feeling lonely. There are supports groups available for spouses; and anybody who's feeling burned out, stressed out, or lonely should check them out.

Barbara McGinnis

If parents think their son's or daughter's pain isn't being taken seriously, they need to speak up. Don't be timid. Don't be mean, either, but don't be intimidated by someone just because they're wearing a white coat. Talk to the nurses, watch the clock, make sure they're following the protocol. But don't start yelling and screaming, because that won't get you anywhere; it'll just antagonize the staff.

7. Exercise: A Key to Pain Relief

This chapter will answer the following questions:

Why is exercise so important for pain relief?

What is the best approach to starting, or returning to, an exercise program for veterans in chronic pain?

What's the best way to treat a sprain or strain to minimize pain and speed healing?

How does exercise benefit amputees?

Benefits of Regular PT

By now you know how much exercise means to me. It was always a key part of my life, but it has been absolutely vital to my recovery and ongoing effort to maintain my health. In the early weeks and months of my recovery, exercise and PT were the only aspects of my life I felt I had any control over. I couldn't handle mental challenges because of my brain injury, but I could still exercise, and I *wanted* to exercise to build my strength and recover faster.

131

Now, four years later, exercise is still critical. Aerobic exercise, like running and bicycling, is important to increase blood flow and oxygen to my limbs. It also helps keep my weight down, which is really important as an amputee because I have to fit into my prosthetic—simply put, if I gain weight, I won't fit.

Basically, exercise helps everything—heart, blood, muscles, and your mind and outlook as well. Let's face it, whether you're a man or a woman, if you maintain your strength and physical shape, you're also going to feel better about yourself, which is part of the overall mission to improve your functioning.

Of course, it's one thing to do PT in boot camp when you have no choice, and quite another when you're back at home, in pain, and maybe stressed out by children, a job, or other complications. It's tough enough for perfectly healthy civilians to carve out time for regular exercise; it's even more challenging when you are in pain from your wounds, when even simple movements like walking and changing position hurt. But here's the irony: the folks for whom exercise is most difficult are the ones who stand to benefit the most from doing it.

Exercise not only keeps you healthy, it will relieve your pain over time. Weight-bearing and cardiovascular exercise strengthens your heart, lungs, bones, and muscles. Physical activity protects against falls and bone fractures— especially important if you are an amputee. Research also suggests that exercise may help control joint swelling and pain caused by arthritis.

I also believe you can "get more bang for your buck" from exercise if you do it with others. I've mentioned before that my closest buddies are the guys I train and race with on Team Semper Fi. I also train with Andrea every chance I get, and that's a real strong, ongoing connection between us. By incorporating friends or family members into your exercise routine, you can build the relationships that support your emotional health, which will, in turn, support your physical health.

Here's a summary of what exercise can do for you:

✪ Release endorphins, which block pain and help alleviate anxiety and depression.

✪ Build strength, which reduces the load on your bones and cartilage and can alleviate pain.

✪ Increase your flexibility, which can also ease pain.

✪ Improve your sleep quality, by slowing the release of stress hormones.

✪ Boost your energy level.

✪ Help you maintain a healthy weight, which can reduce stress on your joints—yet another effective way to relieve chronic pain.

✪ Enhance your mood and self esteem, which will help ward off depression.

✪ Protect your heart and blood vessels, to lower the risk of high blood pressure, diabetes, heart attack, and stroke.

You may find it helpful to work with an exercise physiologist (EP), especially in the start-up phase of a course of physical training. EPs work in wellness or fitness centers, as well as certain clinical settings, such as rehabilitation centers or hospitals. They can help you assess your functional abilities, such as your level of cardiovascular conditioning. They can also tailor the types and intensities of exercise to meet your particular needs. An exercise physiologist may be a member of your pain management team, providing the rest of the team with regular reports on your progress.

Getting Started

You've probably heard this already, but it's important to say it at the outset here: Don't begin an exercise program without first talking to your doctor. This is particularly important if you've been wounded in any serious way, or have a chronic condition such as diabetes or high blood pressure. Your doctor or physical therapist can guide you toward exercise that is appropriate for your level of conditioning, your range of motion, and your state of healing. If you are in pain, you may be worried that exercise will make the pain worse, or that you might injure yourself. That was definitely true for me, and for a while it prevented me from making progress. I was really scared I would hurt myself or end up back in the excruciating pain I felt early on. What I discovered, instead, was that pushing myself a bit, facing my fear, and exercising hard actually reduced my pain in the long run. Okay, I admit, sometimes now I overdo it and have to use take ibuprofen for a few days. Overall, though, I'm totally convinced that my overall pain is less because I exercise. Plus, I sleep better, and

I'm more likely to eat in a healthy way. I just feel better. Period.

Of course, if you're in severe pain, you have to gain some control over it before you start any serious exercise program. A good slogan to follow is: "Start low, go slow." That means starting with low weights, fewer repetitions, and shorter distances, and staying within your limits until you're really ready to move on. As I've said repeatedly, many service men and women are used to pushing their bodies, hard. Please keep in mind, as I've said, that if you have been seriously wounded, you will be deconditioned to one extent or another. Your brain may remember what you used to be capable of but your body will not be up to that level of performance—and you can hurt yourself, make things worse, if you don't take it slow.

When you are considering what type of exercise to do, it's a good idea to begin by thinking about what you actually enjoy doing. You're more likely to stick with an exercise program if it's fun or pleasurable for you in some way. Some people, for example, love gyms and the whole indoor workout culture that goes with it. Other people don't like gyms at all and prefer outdoor exercise such as running, biking, walking, or climbing.

Most exercise programs involve three components:

- ✪ Aerobic exercise raises your heart and breathing rates and sustains that level for at least 20 to 30 minutes.

- ✪ Strength training uses dumbbells, resistance bands, body weight, strength training machines, or improvised weights.

✪ Stretching, either before or after exercising, increases flexibility and lowers the risk of strains, sprains, and other types of injury.

Aerobic Exercise

During aerobic exercise, you repeatedly work large muscles in your arms, legs, and hips, and you breathe faster and more deeply. This maximizes the amount of oxygen in your blood. Your heart beats faster, which increases blood flow to your muscles and back to your lungs. Your small blood vessels expand to deliver more oxygen to your muscles and to carry away waste products, such as carbon dioxide and lactic acid. Aerobic exercise is also the type of exercise that releases **endorphins** (strength training generally doesn't do this).

Aerobic exercise lowers your risk of many conditions, including obesity, heart disease, high blood pressure, type-2 diabetes, stroke, and osteoporosis. Research also shows that it's the *amount* of exercise you do, not the *intensity* that makes the difference. You don't need to sweat buckets and feel as if you're about to pass out, in other words. Doing 30 minutes of moderate exercise is much more beneficial for your body than an intense 10-minute workout.

Strength Training

Many people find that combining some kind of strength training with a program of aerobic exercise improves their endurance and overall fitness level. A regular strength training program can reduce your body fat, increase your lean muscle mass, and help you burn calories more efficiently. It's particularly important that amputees keep up or develop their core strength. By "core strength" I mean the set of internal muscles that stabilize the spine and pelvis and extend the length of the torso. It includes the abdominal and back muscles, as well, but those

Endorphins: A group of hormones released in the brain by stress, pain, or hard exercise. Endorphins that reduce the sensation of pain and boost mood.

are less important than the interior muscles. Many people don't know about these muscles and how important they are, but any plan of strength training should include them. All reputable gyms will have trainers on staff who can teach you some specific exercises to tone and strengthen your core muscles.

Strength training can be done at home or in the gym using the following methods:

✪ Body weight: You can do many exercises with little or no equipment, using only your body weight: push-ups, pull-ups, abdominal crunches, and leg squats.

✪ Resistance bands: Elastic bands of different strengths (usually, in different colors) are inexpensive and versatile tools for doing resistance exercises.

✪ Free weights: Barbells and dumbbells are classic strength training tools. You can also use homemade weights—for example, a plastic soft drink bottle filled with water or sand.

✪ Weight machines: Most fitness centers offer various resistance machines. If you can afford it, you might want to invest in weight machines for home use.

Stretching

Most aerobic and strength training programs inherently cause your muscles to contract and flex. Stretching those muscles after your workout will help prevent and relieve pain and lower your risk of injury. Stretching can also improve the range of motion in your joints, improve your posture, and help relieve stress.

There is ongoing debate about whether stretching before or after exercise is preferable. Scientific data support both camps, so the choice is up to you. On one point, however, everyone agrees: stretching muscles when they're cold raises your risk of injury—notably, pulled muscles. So if you stretch before your workout, take it slow and easy. Alternatively, if you plan to stretch only after your workout, begin the exercise slowly, with more reps and low power to allow your muscles to warm up before you pick up the pace or intensity. When I'm biking I do this by using a low gear for the first 10 minutes or so and "spinning" at high reps.

Here are other tips on stretching:

✪ Feel the pull, not pain. If a stretch hurts, you've gone too far. Back off until you feel no pain, then hold.

✪ Hold each stretch for at least 30 seconds. Muscle tissue takes time to relax and lengthen. Thirty seconds can seem like a long time, so keep an eye on the clock or your watch.

✪ Don't bounce. When you bounce during a stretch you may cause small rips in the muscle that can leave behind scar tissue, which just makes the muscle even less flexible.

✪ Don't hold your breath while you're stretching. Breathe in as you begin a stretch and out as you release it, or vice versa, whichever works for you. Just keep breathing.

Yoga

A form of exercise that deserves attention here is the ancient East Indian discipline of yoga. Yoga teaches balance and flexibility, and draws your attention to breathing and the effect of your mind on your body. There are different forms of yoga but they all involve numerous body positions, called "poses," breathing techniques, relaxation, and sustained concentration or meditation. The poses are designed to improve posture though stretching, toning, and strengthening the muscles, joints, and the spine.

During yoga practice, focus is maintained on regular, deep, conscious breathing. This helps to calm the mind and relax the body. Most types of yoga encourage practitioners to seek a calm, quiet place inside themselves, a kind of refuge or "safe zone" where they can go during times of stress, pain, or the need for restoration.

Yoga is one of the most widely used complementary health techniques. A 2002 survey found that about 15.2

million adults in the United States alone have used yoga to help improve their health. In addition to its potential value for people in chronic pain, yoga may help with other health conditions such as anxiety disorders or stress, asthma, high blood pressure, and depression. Admittedly, yoga isn't as "macho" as pumping iron or sweating on a treadmill, but you might be pleasantly surprised at how much yoga adds to those more hard-core types of exercise. The Exit Wounds website has additional helpful information about yoga.

Sprains and Strains

If you exercise regularly—even if you don't intentionally push yourself or engage in higher-risk activities such as skiing or rock climbing—you're likely at some point to overdo it. A "pulled muscle" is a strain, which occurs when a muscle or tendon is stretched or torn. A sprain happens when you overstretch or tear a ligament, the tough tissue that connects bone to bone. Minor sprains and strains are usually treated at home; but the way you treat them can make a big difference in how fast they heal and how quickly the pain goes away.

There are four steps recommended for dealing with a minor strain or sprain. Use the RICE acronym to remember them:

Rest
Ice
Compression (only possible on certain joints, such as ankles and wrists)
Elevation

VOICES OF SURVIVAL

Bob Nylen served in the First Air Cavalry during the Vietnam War. In 1968, he was shot in his right thigh, had fragments from an RPG (rocket-propelled grenade) embedded in his lower legs, and lost his right eardrum in an explosion from a piece of dynamite wrapped in bamboo.

Bob was also exposed to high levels of Agent Orange, the defoliant that was used liberally in the jungles in the area where he served, near the Ho Chi Minh Trail. He suspects, but cannot prove, that this exposure led to the colon cancer he was diagnosed with in 2004. He underwent radiation
and chemotherapy, and then a five-hour surgery. Although these treatments were successful, he subsequently suffered from pain, both in the hospital and after he was discharged.

"My stomach wall hurt where an eight-inch incision cut muscles," he says. "My butt hurt, too. Just sitting down hurt. Standing hurt. Walking hurt. As someone who had run, played ball, biked, chain-sawed, or did something else strenuous every day of my adult life, it was troubling to find that a flight of steps wiped me out."

Bob says he tried every pill and palliative his doctors offered, but no drug eradicated the pain. Then his wife, Kit, suggested he see a local acupuncturist.

"My pain shrank," he says. "I felt better! The pain didn't disappear, but it hid for a while."

He also took up yoga and meditation, both of which, he says, felt familiar because they involved some of the skills he had learned in the military.

"I began to remember how tranquil I had felt while standing at attention, facing left, facing right," he says.

(continued)

(*Voices of Survival continued*)

"Yes, I already knew yoga, in my bones and sinews! I knew how to hold a pose, quietly. It's all good. The Zen of the parade grounds has its place in the pantheon of self-help."

Bob is combining his use of Eastern techniques with a synthetic morphine delivered through his skin via a patch.

"I'm feeling better," he says. "I'm cutting back on my Oxy-drugs. My body feels like an old summer camp, my plumbing creaking and clanking as it comes back to life following a dormant winter. My new pains are the tolerable pains of healing."

Prompt application of an ice pack on the affected area has been shown to significantly decrease healing time. The cold causes blood vessels to constrict, which reduces swelling and possibly triggers the release of pain-producing compounds from injured tissues. Apply ice or cold for 15 to 20 minutes, then let the area warm up naturally. Repeat every hour as needed to reduce swelling and pain. Caution: Don't put the ice pack directly on the skin; wrap it in a towel or cloth.

After two days, you can switch to heat, because by then swelling should be controlled. Heat opens blood vessels, which can help flush the affected area with blood and oxygen, which can facilitate healing.

You can also use an NSAID pain medication such as ibuprofen to relieve the pain of a strain or sprain. NSAIDs may be preferable to acetaminophen because they have an anti-inflammatory effect, to help reduce swelling.

Exercise after Amputation

Exercise for amputees is itself a major topic of discussion, so I'll cover it only briefly here and direct you to the Exit Wounds website, where you'll find excellent, more detailed information. In short, know that you don't have to run races, like I do—though I find doing so helps keep me motivated to train and work out. Doing any kind of regular workout will provide all the benefits of exercise and—just as important—will improve your prosthetic performance and the health of the remaining portion of a limb.

If you have a lower-limb prosthesis, here are some key points to consider as you work up to aerobic exercise:

✪ Develop a good sense of balance over both your feet.

✪ Maintain equal weight-bearing through both lower limbs.

✪ Learn to use your muscles in the socket, your knee, and your hip quickly and efficiently, because timing is everything.

✪ Keep your body weight over your prosthetic limb long enough to fully deflect the prosthetic foot for maximum "energy release."

✪ Practice moving in multiple directions with your prosthesis, encouraging use of your muscles in a variety of situations.

Patience is key: It takes time to learn to use any prosthesis, and practice makes perfect! Once you learn to let your prosthesis work for, instead of against, you, your life will become much more rewarding.

The Best Medicine

I hope this chapter has convinced you of the benefits of regular exercise, especially if you're in chronic pain. A good program, started slowly and guided by your doctor or other healthcare worker, can do more for your health, your mood, your recovery, and your pain control than any other single component of care including medication. Yes, medications can be invaluable, even indispensable. As I've said, you need to bring your pain under at least partial control before you can begin to exercise regularly and effectively. With that piece in place, you can begin to enjoy the many ways exercise improves all aspects of your being—physical, emotional, mental, even spiritual. No pill or device can do that. You owe it to yourself to take full advantage of the healing powers of exercise!

THE FAMILY JOURNEY

✪ Recognize that exercise for veterans who were wounded or who are dealing with pain is not a luxury; it's a critical part of their recovery and ongoing ability to function. Encourage them to take the time they need to exercise.

✪ If possible, exercise with the service member in your life. It can be a great way to bond and strengthen your relationship.

✪ If a family member has decided to introduce a healthy diet as part of his or her overall program of exercise, encourage everyone in the household to eat the same way. It's much easier to stick to a healthy diet when everyone in the family shares the same meals.

✪ Remind your loved one that even if they don't feel like exercising at first, they will feel better once they start, and *much* better after they've finished. Praise them for sticking with it!

Andrea

I try to support Derek's exercising and training as much as I can, because if that's his way of relieving his anxiety and dealing with stress, then that's a healthy way of doing it. It's better than abusing drugs or alcohol. So I think it's fine for a veteran to exercise a lot, unless it's affecting the marriage. Then maybe you'd need to take it down a notch and find a compromise. But, personally, I don't want Derek to ever stop exercising because it helps him so much.

Barbara McGinnis

One thing family members can to do support a wounded veteran is to exercise with them somehow. Derek and I have done several walks sponsored by a local hospital. I wasn't exactly in shape at first, but Derek pushed me to do them. First we did only 1 mile; next it was 3 miles. It was so cool doing something with the family, something healthy.

David McGinnis

Derek is talking about getting back into snowboarding. We'll make it happen. I know the prosthetist will work with him to get a leg that works for 'boarding. So it looks like it'll really happen, and I'll take a day off from work in a second to do it with Derek.

8. Treating the Emotional Wounds of War

The chapter will answer the following questions:

Why do some people resist getting help for mental or
  emotional difficulties?
What is a "confiding relationship" and why is having one
  important to healing?
What sorts of treatments exist for mental or emotional
  difficulties?
What are some ways to rekindle and revive a sex life that
  has waned because of chronic pain?
What role does spirituality play in reducing pain and
  healing mental and physical wounds?
What is "resilience" and how does it differ from classical
  strength?

Pain Changes Everything

From reading my story in Chapter 1 you know how many
challenges I faced during my recovery that had nothing

directly to do with my body or physical pain. This drives home the point I keep making that pain ripples through all parts of your life and the lives of those around you. I went through a profound depression. Sometimes I was overly anxious or keyed up. And I had all kinds of emotional reactions to the adjustments I had to make as the result of my injuries.

Even today I continue to deal with emotional, nonphysical issues. For example, in the weeks leading up to the fourth anniversary of when I was blown up, I was in a pretty foul mood. I was quick to anger, moody, unhelpful, or downright rude to Andrea, and a general pain in the ass. Thing is, I didn't realize at the time that my bad mood had anything to do with the anniversary. In fact, I didn't even think I *was* in a bad mood; I thought it was other people who were the problem, or that other issues in my life were causing me to be angry or irritable or whatever.

It was only after I went for some personal counseling later in November that I could look back and recognize what had been going on, see the powerful ongoing effect that my injuries could have on my psyche. Those insights really taught me to step back, accept responsibility for my behavior, go back and work things out with Andrea, and get moving forward again with my life.

This is just one small example of the larger issue of what I call the "invisible wounds" that so many returning service men and women have. Although these wounds cannot be seen, like a scar or a lost limb, they can be as painful and disabling as any mortar wound or shrapnel injury.

Likewise, treating invisible wounds can be just as challenging as treating chronic pain. As tricky and complicated as physical pain can be, addressing it at least involves somewhat tangible factors—nerves, brains, limbs, and tissue. But emotional pain? Depression? Post-deployment stress reactions? For many reasons, these can be more difficult to treat than the physical pain that often is the root of the problems. That means it's even more important not to ignore them and to seek help sooner rather than later. Because, just like physical pain, untreated mental and emotional problems usually get worse over time.

Fortunately, as for physical pain, there many ways to treat, heal, and overcome emotional pain and wounds, and I'll review the major options in this chapter. To begin, however, I have to state that it's up to yo to seek out these options. *You have to take the first step.* You have to ask for help and look for answers. This isn't always—or maybe ever—easy, especially for veterans. In some quarters, there remains a stigma about seeking help for mental conditions such as depression, anxiety reactions, sexual problems, or relationship difficulties. Actually, there's something of a stigma in the military about asking for help of any kind. On duty or in combat, weakness is seen as bad; strength and self-reliance as good. Even off duty, asking for help, as rational and healthy as that is, may be perceived by some as weakness. Add to that the very human reluctance to face a mental or emotional problem and you've got a high barrier that many veterans have to overcome before they can make even the first move to getting help.

Fortunately, there is growing awareness in the military that addressing mental health issues is important, that mental health services must be provided, and that commanders need to convey the common-sense idea that everyone has these kinds of problems now and then, and that getting help for them is a sign of strength, not weakness. It's even more critical to seek help if you're in chronic pain, because life difficulties can really get in the way of your progress.

One thing that might make it easier for you to seek out help is to know that counseling of various sorts is usually covered by medical insurance programs. The resources are there. You just have to ask for them.

POSTTRAUMATIC STRESS AND POSTTRAUMATIC STRESS DISORDER (PTSD)

If you've seen combat, you may have been on missions that exposed you to horrible and life-threatening experiences. You may have been shot at, seen a buddy shot or killed, or watched innocent people die. After experiencing these kinds of events, nearly everyone will feel some degree of posttraumatic stress as the result of the continuous and heightened state of arousal in the nervous system. Posttraumatic stress, which includes symptoms such as intrusive thoughts and memories, sleep problems, and anxiety, is a normal human reaction to abnormal circumstances and events.

Sometimes the symptoms of posttraumatic stress do not fade. Instead, they become entrenched and/or amplified to a degree that they begin to seriously disrupt one's life, at which point the person is said to have posttraumatic stress disorder. Why some people experience PTSD and others don't is not known. The important thing is to understand that this disorder is tightly linked to chronic pain, as I described earlier in the book. Having PTSD can raise your risk of suffering chronic pain and can make treating it more difficult.

According to the U.S. Department of Veterans Affairs, about 6 to 11 percent of veterans of OEF and between 12 and 20 percent of OIF veterans have been diagnosed with PTSD. The actual figures are almost certainly higher, however, because many veterans don't admit to their symptoms or may not even realize that what they're experiencing are symptoms of PTSD. (One potential cause of PTSD is sexual abuse that occurs within the military. This source of PTSD is only recently beginning to get the attention it deserves, and the service members who have endured the abuse are finally beginning to get much-needed support.)

PTSD is a type of anxiety disorder. It can happen to anyone who has been through a traumatic event during which they saw horrible things, made them fear for their lives, or feel helpless. The powerful emotions caused by the event produces changes in the brain that may result in PTSD.

PTSD symptoms usually emerge soon after the traumatic event, but it's just as likely they won't begin to occur until months or even years later. They also may come and go over many years. If you have symptoms that last longer than four weeks, cause you great distress, or interfere with your work or home life, you probably have PTSD.

There are four major symptoms of PTSD:

✪ Reliving the event. This may happen in the form of nightmares or flashbacks; it may also display as hypersensitivity to loud noises.

✪ Avoidance of situations or people that trigger memories of the traumatic event, or keeping busy to avoid thinking or talking about the event.

✪ Emotional numbing, feeling distant from loved ones, or loss of interest in activities you used to enjoy.

✪ Feeling keyed up, jittery, or always on alert and on the lookout for danger (often referred to as "hyperarousal").

Treating PTSD can be very challenging—it's difficult to confront painful memories and to open up about your feelings. Living with PTSD is almost always harder—on you and on those around you. The good news is that many treatments are available to help you get better.

Later in this chapter I'll talk about cognitive-behavioral therapy (CBT), a type of counseling that appears to be very effective for treating PTSD. There are also various types of cognitive behavioral therapies, such as cognitive therapy and exposure therapy. A similar kind of treatment, called eye movement desensitization and reprocessing (EMDR), is also used for PTSD. Certain medications may be effective, as well. The key, as with physical pain, is to seek help as soon as possible. Talk to your doctor, a counselor, or anyone you trust. Remember: PTSD is nothing to be ashamed of, and you don't have to "tough it out." The brain changes that occur as the result of trauma are as real as any other kind of wound, and they can happen to anybody, even the strongest military warriors.

Besides, leaving PTSD untreated is going to get in the way of you becoming the man or woman you want to be. I've seen this happen all too often, and it's a tragedy, particularly when children are involved. You can't be a good father or mother when you're battling your demons day and night. Getting help for this very common problem can be the key that unlocks the door to many other positive changes in your life!

Survivor Guilt

As I mentioned earlier in the book, survivor guilt is a mental condition that occurs when a person perceives himself or herself to have done wrong, or feels guilty because he or she survived a traumatic event. I have experienced this myself, and it has been both a positive and negative force in my life. Much of my depression, drive, devotion, and anxiety comes from survivor guilt, and I believe it deeply affects other returning combat veterans as well. Physical pain of course increases these feelings, and exacerbates emotional pain as well.

Daily I ask myself the question: "With the seriousness of the injuries I sustained, why am I alive? Why did friends of mine die and I live? Why do others have worse injuries than I? Why was I allowed to see? Why am I blessed to be a father? Why was I able to overcome my pain? Why am I able to cope with a brain injury?" These questions and others haunt me, and I believe they help push me. I believe that these types of questions are also asked by nearly every service member who stays on the battlefield after a friend or fellow service member has been killed or injured. Thoughts like, "I was sitting in that seat yesterday, why I am I alive today?" or thoughts about the families, spouse, or children of a wounded or killed service member. Service members revisit these thoughts daily while still in the field facing the next mission. Still to this day I cannot pick up the phone and call the families of the people I served with who died.

I deal with survivor guilt by living my life as a tribute to those who no longer can. I reflect that if those who died in battle were given a chance to come back for a month, they would do all they could to enjoy everything possible on earth. They would finish their goals, run triathlons, influence their children, help other like-minded service members find peace and solace. I was given a second chance at life as a survivor and am trying to fulfill what others who died cannot.

Confiding Relationships

At the heart of most healing from the emotional wounds of combat (depression, anxiety, or stress responses) is to open up to someone about these issues. Remember the

VOICES OF SURVIVAL

For Sergeant Lawrence Pittman, a mishap during a routine exercise marked the beginning of a new phase in his military life, one defined by injury, pain, and the ongoing efforts to treat them both.

"It started four years ago when I was in Free-Fall School," Pittman recalls. "I had a piece of loose equipment in the groin area of my suit, and when I deployed, the parachute strap caught in the piece of loose equipment. The result was soft tissue contusions and partially torn muscles in my groin area."

Pittman's pain started immediately. Six months after his injury, he underwent surgery to deaden the nerves in his spermatic cord, but the operation left him with increased sensation and more pain. Determined to find relief, Pittman tried a variety of medications and shots before having a spinal cord stimulator implanted.

"I'd say the stimulator reduced my pain 40 to 50 percent," Pittman says. "I was able to leave the wheelchair that I had been in for two years. I walk with a cane now, and I get around pretty well."

Pittman is still on active duty. He says that his ongoing journey with pain is hard, but he tries to remain positive and has learned to rely on the support of loved ones to stay centered.

"I suffer from depression because it's hard to adjust to not being able to do the things I used to do, whether it's jumping out of airplanes, running, or just being the one leading others in activities," explains Pittman. "So I

(*continued*)

(Voices of Survival continued)
stay as busy as I possibly can and keep my mind occupied.
Fortunately, I have a wonderful family—my wife, a son, and
two daughters—that helps me out when I'm having a bad
day. They keep me going and keep me motivated."

phrase I used earlier: "Revealing is healing?" Well, it's a
critical concept here—though, like most bumper-sticker
slogans, easier said than done. You have to ask: Who can
you reveal your innermost fears to, or share your most
wrenching combat experiences with? Who do you know
that can handle that kind of raw personal truth? Who
can you trust to keep things private? Who will understand you—and not judge you—at that deep level of
honesty?

I can't answer those questions for you. All I know for
sure is you need to answer them for yourself: find that person, or those people, in your life. At least one. If you're
lucky, you will have more than one. If no one comes to
mind, you need to cultivate one, perhaps with a professional. For each of us, there are precious few people we
can tell everything to, be utterly and completely honest
with, and who will understand and accept without judgment all we have to say. They are, literally, precious, as
they can be essential to your healing, your recovery, and
your future personal development. These special relationships are called "confiding relationships" in the jargon of
psychotherapy.

Often, people automatically assume that their confiding relationship needs to be with their spouse or partner.

Turns out, that's not the case. Let's be honest: one of the more vexing things about life can be your relationship with your spouse or partner! It's usually easier, and feels safer, to be totally straight with a person you don't live with, are not sleeping with, raising children with, and managing personal finances with.

All that matters is that you identify at least one person with whom you can talk about anything, admit everything, and reveal all the sides of your personality—the good, the bad, and the ugly. Why is this so important? Why is complete candor so healing? Nobody really knows. Undoubtedly, there's something therapeutic in releasing pent-up tension, in the comfort that comes from dropping the masks we all wear from time to time. The poet Walt Whitman wrote in *Song of Myself*: "I am large. I contain multitudes." Talking about your life in the context of a confiding relationship can give voice to these "multitudes." And from that experience comes insight, new perspective, and healing.

Treatment Options for Emotional Wounds

As I noted at the beginning of this chapter, problems with mood, emotions, or relationships can be treated in numerous ways by various types of healthcare professionals. There are many kinds of "talk therapy" alone, for example. And this isn't about laying on a couch and talking about how your mother treated you as a child. Modern talk therapy—such as I used at various times during my recovery—is much more akin to private coaching. You work with a skilled consultant to learn ways to cope, resolve, or solve a particular problem in your life. The emphasis is on dealing with current issues. Of course, some here-and-now problems do have roots in the past, and it can be very helpful to better understand those roots, but that is generally not the focus. Rather, it's to gain greater insight about yourself, who you really are, why you respond the way you do to people and events around you, and how you can learn new, more effective ways to cope with challenging situations.

Stress, anxiety, or depression also involve your brain. Some veterans have actual physical damage to the brain, such as the traumatic brain injury I suffered. Even in the absence of this type of damage, however, who we are as individuals and how we respond to others has everything to do with how our brains function. Being depressed, or anxious, or experiencing combat-related stress reactions all can change the way your brain works—and not for the better. That's why it can sometimes help to use medications that buffer stress,

TYPES OF MENTAL HEALTH PROFESSIONALS

Psychiatrists are medical doctors (MDs) with additional training in mental illnesses. They are usually the only mental health providers who can prescribe medications.

Psychologists have a doctoral degree (PhD, or PsyD) and special training in mental illnesses. They often work with MDs who can prescribe medications.

Clinical social workers have at least a master's degree in social work. They deal most often with family or interpersonal problems.

Counselors assist people with many types of problems, including mental health issues. They may not have formal training in psychotherapy. Pastoral counselors, for example, use their religious traditions to help people deal with personal problems.

calm anxiety, and/or boost energy and outlook. The subject of medications used to treat emotional problems is much too large to cover in detail here, so again I direct you to the excellent information available on the Exit Wounds website. My purpose here is to briefly introduce you to the types of psychotherapies that can be helpful in dealing with the emotional challenges that often accompany chronic pain. Interestingly, some forms of psychotherapy have been shown in scientific studies to be just as effective as medications for helping people address problems of mood, anxiety, or stress.

The words "counseling," "therapy," and "psychotherapy" are often used to describe the same process. Whichever term you use, counseling involves a series of discussions with a trained professional who can guide you in identifying your feelings or problems, encourage you to talk about them, and help you find ways to cope with or, ideally, solve them. You can do counseling and therapy individually, with another person, with a family, in a group, or a combination of these. Therapists working with couples often see the individuals separately, as well as together. When working with families, they may see each member one at a time, the parents together and/or separately, other combinations of family members, or the whole family together.

Therapy doesn't need to be long term—a great deal of progress can be made during short-term, goal-oriented programs of between 6 and 12 sessions.

Counseling, needless to say, is a highly personal process, and a good match between a counselor or therapist and a client is absolutely critical to its success. As a potential client, the more information you have, the easier

it will be to find the person you feel comfortable working with and can trust. Like medical doctors, therapists
may specialize—treating, say, only women or men, or
children or couples, or groups. They may also have a specialty focus, such as pain, grief, or substance abuse. There
are also many kinds of counseling theories. Some target
personal relationships; others focus on the thought processes that underlie our behaviors; still others focus on
how behavior patterns we learned as children can cause
problems when we are adults. A highly qualified therapist
will know which approach to use to treat a specific problem. When choosing a therapist, the first rule of thumb is
to make sure that he or she is licensed in your state. The
second, and equally important, is to *pay attention to the
way you feel* about any therapist or counselor you con-
sult. Don't stop looking until you find someone who is
genuine, caring, and interested in helping you.

As I mentioned earlier, one type of therapy that has
been shown in many studies to work well for those suffering from PTSD is cognitive-behavioral therapy (CBT).
CBT involves a relatively short series of weekly meetings
with a therapist with the goal of identifying and changing negative or irrational thought patterns that can lead
to dysfunctional behaviors. (The actual number of sessions varies widely and, sad to say, often is influenced
as much by insurance or health plan policies as actual
patient needs.) For instance, you might not realize how
deeply worried you are about injury-related changes in
your physical appearance, and how those worries lead
you to curtail the way you express your affection for your
partner. During CBT, therapists help patients recognize
these kinds of patterns and suggest ways to interrupt or

replace negative or disruptive thinking with more realistic positive attitudes and expectations.

For difficulties with relationships, other types of therapy can be very helpful. Interpersonal therapy is a pragmatic, results-oriented process that typically involves 12 to 16 one-hour sessions. Interpersonal therapy may involve the client's partner as well, in which case it may be called couples therapy.

Family therapy can be extremely valuable when children, teens, or other family members have been affected by the emotional problems of the returning veteran. Family therapy can provide a safe forum where everyone is given the opportunity to speak and be heard. It can be difficult, but also tremendously rewarding.

Group therapy, as I discovered during my recovery time in Texas, can also be very useful. Being with others who understand what you've been through or are currently going through can be comforting, supportive—even fun at times.

Where can you go to find a counselor, therapist, or support group? You can start with your command or installation chaplain if you are on active duty, or go to your local VA or vet center if you're a veteran. These people will be able to suggest counselors who are attuned to military lifestyle issues and are prepared to offer professional assistance. These services are usually free; they are also confidential—unless you are considered to be a danger to yourself or others, in which case, the counselor may be compelled to reveal information to ensure the safety of all concerned. You can also look for counselors and therapists in your local community. As I mentioned earlier, private services may be covered by your insurance (see the resources section for contact information).

Spiritual Healing

In addition to formal or informal counseling or therapy, you might want to consider joining a faith community where you feel comfortable. Many veterans have faced death or been forced to confront their own mortality at an age when their civilian contemporaries see only the endless possibilities in life. Being in the line of fire or coming close to death can be a life-changing experience. It typically forces you to reassess your priorities and values, and to reconsider what gives you meaning or purpose in life. That has certainly been true for me and for a lot of veterans I know. I'm definitely a more spiritual person now than I was before I was injured. For me, it's not about going to church—though we do go as a family most Sundays. It's about being thankful, all the time, for what I have. I'll be driving and see a sunset, and I stop to appreciate it, and thank the Lord for the day. Or I'll be outside playing catch with my boys and take a second to give thanks for that. My faith also helps me control my stress and anxiety: when things go wrong, I do my best to trust that things will work out, and I pray for the strength to help others.

I don't want to sound preachy here—everybody's free to believe, or not believe, what they want. All I'm saying is that, for me and many other veterans, finding some kind of spiritual connection or spiritual community can aid in recovery and in coping with chronic pain. There's something about enduring pain, especially when it seems arbitrary and mysterious and unmanageable, that introduces a spiritual dimension to your life. Pain forces you to confront the randomness and unfairness of life and of war. On the bright side, it can also make you a more compassionate person.

Rekindling Intimacy

One type of invisible wound deserves special attention in this discussion: sexual problems. Often, one of the first casualties of a chronic pain condition is intimacy. Pain itself is a turnoff, needless to say, but the other complications I've been talking about also take their toll. Plus, many of the medications used to treat pain can reduce sex drive and/or sexual response. The common result: a damaged and dysfunctional sex life. Complicating the problem is that few people are willing to talk about it—even to their partners!

You owe it to yourself and your partner to seek ways to regain a level of intimacy—specifically, sexual pleasure. Besides being a natural and healthy part of life, sex can also ease pain by releasing endorphins and lowering stress, as I mentioned earlier in the book. It's crucial, as well, to reconnecting with a partner or spouse and to sustaining closeness and trust.

How you and your partner go about restoring your sexual life will depend on the nature of the wounds suffered by the injured partner. Obviously, the more serious the injury, the more likely it is that one or both of you will have to adjust the way you make love. In fact, intercourse may not even be possible if, for example, the genitals were seriously injured. Still, even in the most extreme cases, it usually is possible to give and receive pleasure in other ways, which provide a form of intimacy that can be just as deep and satisfying as intercourse. By focusing on the intimacy, rather than penetration or intercourse, and broadening your concept of sex, you almost certainly will find satisfaction.

Resilience: A Better Kind of Strength

I want to end my discussion of the emotional dimension of chronic pain by introducing a concept that can help you improve your mental and emotional functioning and protect you from future stresses or trauma. Research in both psychology and neuroscience suggests that people have an innate psychological **resilience**, and that resilience can be strengthened. Resilience is the capacity to maintain, recover, and improve your mental and physical health in the face of challenge. Simply put, you can learn to build your psychological reserves, toughen your physical responses to stress, and become less vulnerable to maladies such as anxiety or depression.

At the core of resilience is flexibility, not rigidity. This is a different kind of strength from what you are probably used to. Resilience implies a capacity to absorb blows, rather than repel them with armor. Resilience also means giving way to the full spectrum of human emotion, from positive to negative, as appropriate to a given situation, so that you don't become stuck in any emotion or fixated on a problem or event.

The idea of resilience isn't exactly new. Lao Tzu, the great Chinese philosopher, wrote some 2600 years ago in the *Tao Te Ching*:

> *Green plants are tender and filled with sap*
> *At their death they are withered and dry*
> *Therefore the stiff and unbending is the disciple*
>   *of death*
> *The gentle and yielding is the disciple of life*

This may sound hopelessly naïve to a service member, a sailor, an airman, or a soldier who has been trained to kill and survive the ravages of war. But Lao Tzu isn't talking about fighting a war; he's talking about living a life. You certainly *do* need "armor" in battle, you *do* need a rigid kind of strength, and you cannot be gentle with an enemy intent on killing you. But you're home now. Switching to a resilient type of strength is going to be far more productive and rewarding than remaining clenched like fist, in a perpetual fighting stance.

How can you become more resilient? Many veterans have already had experiences that can promote resilience. The adage "what doesn't kill you makes you stronger" contains an important element of truth, verified by researchers studying resilience. Many people emerge from a challenge such as the loss of a family member or engaging in combat saying they have gained from their experience. In my own case, I can say that adversity and trauma have produced greater resiliency.

Resilience is the capacity to maintain, recover, and improve your mental and physical health in the face of challenge.

It has also been shown that aerobic exercise can produce effects that mirror those induced by moderate, intermittent stress. For example, physical training programs have been linked to lower baseline physiological arousal rates, quicker return to baseline after stress, improved use of blood sugar, ease of muscle tension, and a reduction in various compounds associated with the fight-or-flight arousal of the nervous system.

My point here is that as you cope with chronic pain and recover your functioning, you should also consider

In the midst of winter, I finally
learned that there was in me an
invincible summer.
—*Albert Camus*

adding as a goal to improve your overall resilience. Of course, it won't be a smooth, uninterrupted process. Life events will happen that sometimes support and occasionally erode resiliency. But by attending to both your physical health and the non-physical issues I've discussed in this chapter, you can make steady progress and reach goals you might not believe are possible now.

THE FAMILY JOURNEY

✪ Encourage a returning service member to seek help with any mental, emotional, or relationship issues that he or she might be having.

✪ Be willing to go with a family member to a counselor or therapist, if he or she requests or suggests doing so.

✪ If a service member joins or attends a spiritual community, go to services with him or her.

Andrea

It's very important to have somebody you can vent to, somebody who can say, "I know exactly what you're going through." I've got a friend whose husband is an above-the-knee amputee like Derek, and we get together all the time and talk about our husbands. It's so important to have that, so you know you're not crazy—somebody who can say, "Oh yeah, my husband does the same thing..."

Don't be afraid to go to a counselor if you need it. I did that when I was pregnant with Ryan, in San Antonio, because I had a really hard time—and I'm not really into counselors—but I was desperate and needed somebody to talk to. I had girlfriends I could talk to, which was good, but sometimes you need a counselor. Now, sometimes it's not a good fit. The counselor I saw there was horrible—I wasn't happy with how he was dealing with me. I went to two sessions and never went again. Before that I'd gone to another counselor in Hawaii during the time when Derek and I were apart, and he was depressed in Bethesda. I was a wreck. This counselor was really great—he helped a lot. So my advice is to try it, and if it's a bad fit, don't continue. Drop 'em and find somebody you like and who listens to you.

Barbara McGinnis

We didn't try to pry anything out of Derek. You can't push it. I instinctively knew he needed to talk to a peer. Sometimes a parent isn't the closest one to a child, or the best person for them to talk to about personal things. Sometimes it's a best buddy, or an uncle. If you, as a parent, are concerned about something but don't feel comfortable bringing it up with your child, you should talk to somebody else who is close and ask that person talk to your son or daughter.

David McGinnis

You need to talk about things in order to heal, no matter what the issue is. If you vent, you feel better. Sometimes veterans hold back because they want to talk to somebody who understands. I get that. There are some things that a nonmilitary parent just won't understand. Then they need to find other veterans to talk to who have been through the same kinds of things.

9. Getting the Help You Deserve

This chapter will answer the following questions:

How can you get the best care from providers and
  healthcare systems?
What are recovery coordinators and what do they do?
To what kinds of medical benefits are veterans entitled?
How does the military determine level of benefits for those
  who were severely wounded in combat?
How does the Combat-Related Special Compensation
  process work?

Mastering the System

Throughout this book I've urged you to learn as much as
you can about whatever issues you face so that you'll be
more in control of your situation and raise your chances of
recovering your health and functioning. That means learning about your body, about pain, and about your various
treatment options. But there's another—and equally important—subject area that any wounded service member needs

to master: the military and veterans healthcare bureaucracies. That's right—there are two bureaucracies to deal with. The Department of Defense medical system is different from—and until recently separate from—the medical system created and maintained by the Veterans Administration. Lately there have been increasing efforts to get these two systems to work more seamlessly together, but there is still a long way to go. It is also true that many veterans seek care at civilian medical centers in addition to or instead of the military and VA healthcare systems. Learning about your rights and eligibility for coverage and care are essential to your recovery and well-being.

It's vitally important that you or a family member who is working on your behalf not give up in the face of complicated rules, overstressed administrators, or policies that don't seem to make sense. I doubt I'd be here today writing this book and living my life with Andrea and my boys if I hadn't done my homework back when I was at Walter Reed and Bethesda Naval Hospital and then maneuvered my way into a transfer to Brooke Army Medical Center in Texas. That didn't just happen. I *made* it happen. I made it happen not by giving in to hysterics or threatening lawsuits or aggressive confrontations; I did it by learning the rules of the systems, following the chain of command, and being assertive—respectfully assertive—at every step of the way.

This is not an easy path, I know. Sometimes I got so mad or frustrated I wanted to just quit. But don't give up and check out of the system, or you will miss out on a huge amount of assistance and services you may be entitled to and that could speed your recovery and support you and those you love in the years to come.

The military and veterans healthcare systems are vast, and the doctors, nurses, administrators—practically everyone—is over-burdened, short on time, and often, as a result, short on patience. That means you sometimes have to be the "squeaky wheel" to get the attention and care you deserve. In this chapter I'll talk about the most effective ways to go about getting the best possible medical care and pain treatment. I'll also review the types of medical benefits for which you may be eligible. (For more information on veterans benefits visit www.va.gov or the *American Veterans' and Servicemembers' Survival Guide,* which is available online at www.veteransforamerica.org).

Using a Recovery Coordinator

When a service member has been seriously wounded, one of the first administrative things that happens is to be assigned to a recovery coordinator at the military hospital where recovery takes place. Coordinators are part of a new program designed to orchestrate care in both the military and civilian healthcare systems. Your coordinator can be a key resource. He or she will work with the doctors, nurses, social workers, and service-specific program staff to create your recovery plan. This plan will guide you as you go about identifying, applying for, and receiving all the benefits and compensation you're entitled to. Depending on where you are being cared for, your recovery coordinator may be available in person or via phone and e-mail.

Working with Healthcare Providers

As you interact with the various medical providers in the healthcare system, keep the following questions in mind:

✪ Are your providers clearly communicating medical information to you?

✪ Are they giving you enough information so that you can make informed choices about your treatment?

✪ Do they give you referrals to specialists when you ask for them?

✪ Are your own suggestions and inquiries regarding your care treated with respect? Are your questions answered to your satisfaction?

✪ Are your requests for second opinions granted quickly and without resistance?

If the answer to any of these questions is no, it's time to think about finding another provider. Yes, that is a hassle; and no, you shouldn't have to do it. But as in the rest of life, some relationships work out better than others; some people are a better "fit" for your particular needs, style, or personality; and sometimes everyone is better off by separating and moving on. If you have made a good-faith effort to work with your providers but things aren't working out after a matter of weeks or months, look elsewhere.

Don't forget, though, you have responsibilities in these various healthcare relationships as well. For starters, come to office visits prepared with information you want explained, or lists of questions you want answered (consider bringing a friend or relative along to take notes). During appointments, ask about *anything* you don't understand, and don't leave until it's clear to you what you are supposed to do after you leave the office. Ask providers to write down any instructions you think you might

---

VOICES OF SURVIVAL

Darisse was an Army helicopter pilot who flew many missions in Iraq. The vibrations from the helicopter, which were transmitted to her spine via the very hard seat, produced low back pain and stiffness during her deployment. The pain progressively worsened, and just before she was to return home she developed "horrible" shooting pain down her left leg.

"I was stationed in a remote location and had no access to Western medical care, so I just sucked it up until I got home," she says.

She was diagnosed as having a herniated disk between two of her lower vertebrae, as well as radiculopathy (pain related to a damaged nerve). She endured a year of conservative therapy: physical therapy, chiropractic care, and 14 different pain management injections, none of which eased the pain.

"You name it, I tried it—epidural injections, facet joint injections, radiofrequency denervations, and selective nerve root injections," she says.

The pain was so unrelenting that Darisse was forced to accept a medical discharge from the Army. In January 2007, she had surgery to repair the herniated disc and relieve the pressure on the nerve root. But because the root had been damaged for so long, she still felt the shooting leg pain, even though the original injury had been fixed.

She landed a job as a sales rep for a veterinary diagnostics company, but the job required a great deal of driving, which aggravated her pain. In October 2007, she

(*continued*)

(*Voices of Survival continued*)
had another surgery to fuse the two vertebrae. Recovery
took two months, and still she had the chronic leg pain.

"I can't begin to explain how frustrating it was to have
gone through all of these treatments and still have debilitating pain," she says. "I once was an active triathlete, and also
enjoyed hiking, mountain biking, snowboarding, and playing basketball. The leg pain turned me into a couch potato
and made me depressed."

Then she found a pain management doctor who suggested a spinal cord stimulator.

"I didn't want to get my hopes up that it would work,"
she says. "I had been through so many procedures with no
results. But the stimulator worked. It was amazing—I ran,
biked, and walked my dogs. The sensation of the stimulator
is so pleasant; it is like getting a leg massage all day. Now
I have hope again that I can be a normal, active, 29-year-old."

forget; or be proactive and bring a notebook and pencil
with you to write them down yourself. (I recommend you
keep one notebook for all your medical appointment notes;
it makes it easier to stay organized.) Another thing: obtain
a copy of all your medical records and keep it updated! If
you have not yet been discharged, be sure to get a certified
copy of your service-related medical records that is properly stamped and signed, prior to your discharge.

If you're having some kind of difficulty, whether it's
the side effect of a medication, an inability to stick to a
treatment plan, a financial problem, or any other concern,
speak up! Your healthcare provider may be able to make
adjustments in your recovery plan that will make things

better. You may, for example, be able to gradually reduce the dosage of the medicine causing unpleasant side effects, or learn about financial aid available through a veteran-related service organization. And on those days you're feeling discouraged or so frustrated you can't remain calm and respectful when dealing with providers or administrators, call on a trusted family member or friend for support. It's important to advocate for yourself, but it's just as important to acknowledge when you need to let somebody else step in and lobby on your behalf.

If you are using—or want to use—some type of complementary or alternative medicine treatment such as acupuncture, it's important to share the information with everyone on your health team. They won't—or shouldn't—take offense if you want to seek care from an alternative healthcare provider, and they can advise you about such things as, for example, interactions between certain herbal products and any traditional medications you might be using.

Service-Connected Disability Compensation

Once your wound has been stabilized—that is, you have healed to the extent possible—you can apply for Service-Connected Disability Compensation. In this process, called the Disability Evaluation System (DES), you follow a formal set of guidelines to determine which benefits you are eligible for and what level of services you will need. DES usually begins when your doctor has determined that you have suffered a permanent or long-lasting effect from a wound, illness, or injury. Note that because every patient and every situation is different, your doctor may delay writing the required narrative summary of your case and referring you to the DES until he or she sees how you respond to treatment and rehabilitation therapy. Your doctor will refer your case only after he or she is satisfied that everything medically possible has been done to improve your condition. The services also generally require doctors to initiate the DES process after a year of treatment for the same injury or illness.

Each branch of military service uses a slightly different method to enter a service member into the DES, and for determining the level of disability. The Army, for instance, uses a physical profile system that measures a soldier's physical limitations in six areas, with a level assignment of between 1 (fully healthy) and 4 (severely limited) in each. If a soldier receives a permanent level 3 or 4 in any area, the doctor is required to recommend that a Medical Evaluation Board (MEB) review the soldier's case. In contrast, in the Navy and Marine Corps, the process begins with the doctor writing a narrative summary; no prior requirements exist. Talk with your chain of command and your doctors to find out how the DES process operates in your branch of the service.

In all branches of the military, a copy of your medical record usually is sent to the nearest designated military treatment facility commander, who assigns a Physical Evaluation Board Liaison Officer (PEBLO) to help guide you through the DES process. Once you have been assigned a PEBLO, a Medical Evaluation Board will review your record to decide whether you meet your service's medical retention standards. Each service has branch-specific rules, but generally the MEB is made up of medical professionals. The PEBLO will compile a packet of information, containing:

✪ Your medical records

✪ Results from tests and medical exams performed for the MEB related to your condition

✪ Letters from your chain of command related to how the injury or illness impacts your duty

✪ Copies of your performance evaluation reports

✪ Other personnel records that the MEB may require

In reviewing your case, the MEB members are responsible for answering the question: "Do you meet the retention standards for your service?" During the review process, they may conclude:

✪ That you meet medical retention standards, and return you to full duty in your current job.

✪ That you meet medical retention standards in another job, and recommend you retrain for that position.

✪ That you do not meet the medical retention standards, in which case they will forward a recommendation to a Physical Evaluation Board (PEB).

This is an important point that can be confusing: the MEB does *not* determine your fitness for duty or level of disability. That determination is made only by the PEB. By the way, this is the kind of thing I was talking about that can trip you up, if you don't do your homework. Fortunately, today, most of what you need to know is available on the

Internet. Using a search engine like Google makes it much easier and faster than in the past to find exactly the information you need. (If you're not familiar with computers or search engines, now's a good time to learn!)

Physical Evaluation Boards usually consist of three people, made up of a mix of military and civilian members, and usually include a line officer and a senior medical officer. Typically, the PEB will meet informally to review your case, and you will not be required to attend. Using the packet developed by the PEBLO during the MEB process, the board will review your medical record, the doctor's narrative summary, your personnel evaluations, and letters from your commander. It will then make a preliminary decision on your case as to whether you are fit or unfit for continued service. The members will rate the severity of any disability you may have, between 0 and 100 percent. They will then decide your disposition: return to duty, separation, or permanent or temporary retirement.

Your PEBLO will notify you of the findings of the informal PEB. At this point, you have to choose between requesting a formal PEB or accepting the informal PEB findings. If you decide you want a formal PEB hearing, you will be allowed to appear before the board to ask them to reconsider their decision. At this time, you may also provide them additional information important to that reevaluation. You also have a right to be represented by legal counsel at the formal PEB. Subsequently, if you disagree with the determination of the formal PEB, you have the right to appeal the decision.

The processes used by both the Department of Defense and the VA to determine disability level are complicated. So if you are thinking of filing a claim for disability compensation, be prepared to dig in and learn as much as you can about these procedures. There is no substi-

tute for knowledge! Start with the information on the Exit
Wounds website. Then talk to other veterans who have
been through the process. A great way to do this is to go to
a meeting of your local VFW or American Legion and ask
around to learn who in the bureaucracy is good to work
with. Talk to your doctor and others on your healthcare
team, too. And if you're confused about anything, keep
asking questions until the answers become crystal clear.

If your combined disability rating is 30 percent or
higher, and your condition is considered stable (meaning
it is unlikely, in your doctor's opinion, that your disability
rating will change within five years), you will be permanently retired for disability. You will then be eligible for
disability retirement pay, access to TRICARE for you and
your dependent family members, access to commissary
and exchange shopping, and all other benefits of regular
military retirement.

Types of Veteran Benefits

Many types of medical benefits are available to veterans.
Which you may be eligible for depends on such things as the
seriousness of your disability, length of service, and the military branch in which you served. Here are the most common
types of medical or health-related benefits (many others,
such as direct disability compensation, exist as well).

Medical Care

The Department of Veterans Affairs (VA) offers medical
care in its nationwide system of medical centers, clinics, rehab centers, and nursing homes. Access to VA medical care

is based on discharge status, length of service, disability rating, and income level. Veterans with service-connected disabilities receive the highest priority at VA medical facilities.

The VA offers a host of special programs for veterans, including:

- ✪ Treatment for Gulf War illness
- ✪ Treatment for PTSD and TBI
- ✪ Services for blind veterans
- ✪ Readjustment counseling
- ✪ Dental care
- ✪ Home healthcare
- ✪ Hearing aids

Caregiver Financial Support

When I was injured I was incredibly fortunate that my parents and other relatives could take weeks of time off from work and fly across the country to be by my side. That's not always possible, for a lot of reasons. In the past, the family members of veterans often were forced to choose between keeping their jobs and providing care for an injured service member. Then, in 2008, Congress passed legislation that allows for payments to caregivers under certain conditions. Under the new rules family members may be eligible for up to 26 weeks of unpaid leave in a one-year period to care for an injured service member. To access this benefit, however, the service member must have a serious injury or illness that occurred in the line of duty; and not all family members are eligible. Spouses, children, parents, and/ or a next of kin are usually covered, if they meet the legal requirements for length of employment at place of work. Other family members may be eligible, in some cases.

Home and Car Adaptation

Veterans and service members with certain service-connected disabilities may be eligible for grants to enable them to adapt their homes or cars to meet their disability requirements.

Community-based Counseling

The VA operates a system of 232 community-based Vet Centers, staffed by small teams of dedicated providers, many of whom are combat veterans themselves. Vet Centers provide individual, group, and family counseling, *free of charge*, to all veterans who served in any combat zone. Here are some of the types of support you will find at Vet Centers:

- Readjustment counseling
- Marriage and family counseling
- Grief counseling
- Assistance with medical referrals and applying for VA benefits
- Employment guidance and referral
- Alcohol and drug abuse counseling
- Counseling and referrals to treat sexual trauma that occurred during service

The great thing about these services is that most of the people providing the support are or have been in the military. Many are former combat veterans themselves, and so understand these issues at a level civilian healthcare professionals simply can't.

Vocational Rehabilitation

The VA offers rehabilitation and employment services to help service members transition out of the military. These programs provide such things as counseling services, education and training, job assistance, and financial aid. To be eligible, you must have a service-connected disability and require vocational rehabilitation in order to find a job. These programs are also available to active-duty service members who are awaiting discharge because of a disability.

If you find you are not getting the care you need through the VA, here are some steps to take:

✪ Talk to your healthcare provider or healthcare team.

✪ Make an appointment with a VA advocate.

✪ Know that legal counsel is available—see the Exit Wounds website for resources.

★★★

I hope this brief review of the bureaucratic and administrative side of getting effective pain treatment and military benefits will encourage you to persevere in your efforts. Yes, the system can be daunting, but I'm here to tell you that it also can be an ally, and will support you, if you make the effort to understand how it works and maintain your determination and poise in the face of the inevitable obstacles you will face.

THE FAMILY JOURNEY

Family members can help in many ways as an injured service member navigates complex medical and military systems:

✪ Offer to research medical care options, online, at libraries, or by phone. Summarize in writing what you learn.

✪ Make a list of all healthcare providers working with the service member, including their contact information: addresses, phone numbers, and e-mail addresses (if available).

✪ Accompany the family member to medical appointments and serve as "secretary"—take notes and make sure previously raised questions are answered fully.

✪ Read about the various benefits and eligibility requirements for medical care—two heads are better than one, in most cases!

✪ Make sure your service member reviews what he or she is eligible for, and understands that other healthcare insurance plans may be important to review and research. These may impact your current military benefits. This might include Medicare, Medicaid, and Social Security benefits.

Barbara McGinnis

Two days after Derek first arrived at Bethesda Naval Hospital a woman came and gave Andrea a book about military benefits for wounded veterans. We started thumbing through the book, learning about what was available. Of course, Andrea and, later, Derek learned that book backwards and forwards. But it was a good thing that we learned something about it, too. I was worried, because I'd heard of Vietnam-era horror stories of veterans who seemed to have no benefits.

David McGinnis

We didn't have to help Derek too much because he was so self-motivated. But if you're not in that position, or you're on your own as a parent or family member, you need to be proactive. Take advantage of all the help that is available for both veterans and family members. Contact the veterans groups in your area. You have to call them—they're not going to come to you. But when you do connect with them, you'll find a big extended family.

Epilogue: A Call to Action

This book has led you from the details of my own story of injury, struggle, and recovery through the many facets of life that are changed or affected by chronic pain to the steps you can take to treat your pain and move beyond it to regain your health and quality of life. Along the way I've repeated a few refrains: advocate for yourself and your needs; don't give up; get help sooner rather than later; ask for help when you need it; and reach out for support and companionship from those around you.

To close, I'd like to touch on another dimension of recovery: the value of becoming an agent for change. Once you have regained your strength and healed from your wounds, you might want to consider—as I have—what you can do for others facing similar challenges. Obviously, this isn't mandatory, and you may decide it's all you can do to manage your own life and that of your immediate family. I understand, believe me. I'm fully aware that being a good father and husband or partner is more than a full-time job! I would, however, just like to plant the seed that there are many, many ways you might want to become involved in the ongoing effort to help other veterans in pain, to raise awareness about pain issues in general, and to help reform and improve both the DOD and VA healthcare systems responses to those in chronic pain. For me, serving as an advocate with the American Pain Foundation has enriched my life tremendously, and has reinforced many of the lessons

I've learned and tried to convey in this book. It's a cliché, I know, but by helping others, usually you help yourself.

Opportunities to make a difference for others are all around you—often, as near as your local hospital, military base, veterans organization, or school. Even volunteering once a month or visiting other wounded veterans who are in recovery can be hugely rewarding.

Here are some other of the many options to consider:

- Participating in online forums such as the APF's PainAid website, where you can share your experiences and offer your support to those in need.

- Educating yourself about pain-related issues and helping to organize efforts or advocate for legislation or other government initiatives that could improve pain care.

- Joining APF's Power Over Pain Action Network and working with other volunteers to improve pain care within your state by speaking out and communicating with state and local officials.

- Giving talks at local schools, religious groups, or community organizations to raise awareness about the needs of wounded veterans.

- Submitting your story to APF's "Voices of Veterans in Pain" website.

- Writing a letter to the editor of your local paper in response to media reports about veterans or the care they receive.

✪ Helping raise money for pain-related organizations such as APF or the Amputee Coalition of America.

These are just a handful of ideas—there's really no limit to the number of ways veterans and their families can help push forward the goals of more timely and effective pain treatments for service members. By getting involved, you'll be joining a movement of thousands, as well as organizations such as APF, which has been serving people in pain since 1997. The APF's mission is to improve the quality of life of people in pain by raising public awareness, providing practical information, promoting research, and advocating to remove barriers and improve access to effective pain management.

Whether or not you choose to get involved in the larger struggle to help those in pain and improve pain treatments, I hope that this book has inspired you, and will serve as a guide to you going forward, no matter where you are in your own struggle with pain. Maybe you're in the earliest phase of recovery—still in a hospital, still facing surgeries to repair your wounds. Perhaps you're in rehabilitation, relearning former skills or learning new ways to cope with the aftermath of a wound. Maybe you're home, "repaired" to the extent possible, but still in pain. Regardless, I am confident that with persistence and the right team of healthcare providers, you will emerge, as I have, from struggle, pain, and frustration, to live a full life once more. I am confident, too, that one day your life will no longer revolve around pain, that you will have regained important functioning, and be able to look around and appreciate—now with a heightened degree of intensity—the ordinary pleasures of life that each day offers.

Resources for Veterans in Pain and Their Families

The resources listed below represent just a sampling of the many available. For more information, visit www.exit-woundsforveterans.org.

> **American Pain Foundation**
> 1–888–615–PAIN (7246)
> www.painfoundation.org

Find a Military or Veterans-Related Organization

> **Amputee Coalition of America**
> 1–888–267–5669
> www.amputee-coalition.org

> **Coalition for Iraq and Afghanistan Veterans**
> www.coalitionforveterans.org
> A national nonpartisan partnership of over 50 organizations committed to working with and on behalf of all military, veterans, families, survivors, and providers to strengthen the existing system of care and support for all those affected by the wars in Iraq and Afghanistan.

> **Coming Home Project**
> www.cominghomeproject.net
> A nonprofit organization devoted to providing compassionate care, support, and stress management tools for Iraq and Afghanistan veterans, their families, and their service providers.

Defense and Veterans Brain Injury Center
1–800–870–9244
www.dvbic.org

Disabled American Veterans (DAV)
1–877–426–2838
www.dav.org

Iraq and Afghanistan Veterans for American
www.iava.org

National Veterans Legal Services Program
202–265–8305
www.nvlsp.org

One Freedom: Strength Through Balance
www.onefreedom.org
One Freedom offers service members, veterans, and military families a powerful framework of education and training that builds strength, resilience, and a clearer understanding of how to maintain balance in the face of military deployments and other lifestyle challenges.

U.S. Department of Veterans Affairs
1–877–222–8387
www.va.gov

Veterans for America
202–483–9222
www.veteransforamerica.org
Note: *The American Veterans' and Servicemembers' Survival Guide* is available free from this organization's website.

Find a Pain Specialist

American Academy of Family Physicians
www.familydoctor.org

American Academy of Nurse Practitioners
202–966–6414
www.aanp.org

American Academy of Pain Management
209–533–9744
www.aapainmanage.org

American Academy of Pain Medicine
847–375–4731
www.painmed.org

American Academy of Physician Assistants
703–836–2272
www.aapa.org

American Board of Pain Medicine
847–375–4726
www.abpm.org

American Medical Association
312–464–5000
www.ama-assn.org

Case Management Resource Guide
800–784–2332
www.cmrg.com

Commission on Accreditation of Rehabilitation Facilities
520–325–1044
www.carf.org

Mayo Clinic Pain Management Center
www.mayoclinic.com

National Hospice and Palliative Care Organization
703–837–1500
www.nhpco.org

Pain.com
www.pain.com/painclinics/default.cfm

Find a Complementary and Alternative Medicine (CAM) Specialist

American Academy of Medical Acupuncture
323–937–5514
www.medicalacupuncture.org

American Association for Naturopathic Physicians
866–538–2267
www.naturopathic.org

American Association of Oriental Medicine
866–455–7999
www.aaom.org

American Chiropractic Association
703–276–8800
www.amerchiro.org

American Holistic Health Association
714–779–6152
www.ahha.org

American Massage Therapy Association
877–905–2700
www.amtamassage.org

American Osteopathic Association
800–621–1773
www.osteopathic.org

American Physical Therapy Association
703–684–APTA (2782)
www.apta.org

Find a Support Group

American Chronic Pain Association
800–533–3231
www.theacpa.org

Caring Connections
800–658–8898
www.caringinfo.org

Family Caregiver Alliance
800–445–8106
www.caregiver.org

Friends' Health Connection
800–48–FRIEND (483–7436)
www.friendshealthconnection.org

National Chronic Pain Society
281–357–4673
http://ncps-cpr.net

National Family Caregivers Association
800–896–3650
www.thefamilycaregiver.org

PainAid
www.painfoundation.org

Pain Connection
301–309–2444
www.pain-connection.org

Well Spouse Association
800–838–0879
www.wellspouse.org

Endnotes

Introduction

Page 8: Tragically, in 2008, 128 service members killed themselves, which is the highest suicide rate since the military began keeping statistics in 1980. Carden, M.J., Suicide Prevention Hotline Saves Veterans' Lives. American Forces Press Service, February 13, 2009. Available at: www.defenselink.mil/news/newsarticle.aspx?id=53091; accessed: 2/25/09.

Page 9: A recent study of soldiers enrolled in VA Polytrauma Centers showed that more than 90 percent have chronic pain, that most have pain in more than one part of the body, and that pain is the most common symptom in returning soldiers. Lema, M.J., testimony on behalf of Pain Care Coalition before the Committee on Veteran's Affairs Health Subcommittee, U.S. House of Representatives, October 4, 2007.

Chapter 2

Page 43: That so many service men and women survive is all the more remarkable because the wounds in OIF/OEF are so often the result of bombs, not bullets—about 65 percent of the roughly 33,000 soldiers wounded to date were injured by IEDs, land mines, or other "blast phenomena." Clark, ME, et al., Pain and combat injuries in soldiers returning from Operations Enduring Freedom and Iraqi Freedom: implications for research and practice. *J Rehabil Res Dev.* 44(2): 179–194, 2007.

Page 43: For example, of the thousands of soldiers, like me, who are wounded by blasts, fully 60 percent suffer traumatic brain injury (TBI)—a rate much higher than in previous wars: Gawande, A., Casualties of War—military care for the wounded of Iraq and Afghanistan. *New England Journal of Medicine*, 351(24): 2471–2475, 2004.

Page 52: A recent report found that Reserve and National Guard soldiers who were deployed and had combat exposure were significantly more likely to begin heavy weekly drinking and binge drinking upon their return, compared to Reserve/National Guard members who did *not* deploy. Jacobson, I.G., Ryan, M.A.K., Hooper, T.I., et al., Alcohol Use and Alcohol-Related Problems Before and After Military Combat Deployment. JAMA 300(6): 663–675, 2008.

Chapter 3

Page 60: About 76 million people suffer from this kind of pain [chronic pain] in the United States alone: National Center for Health Statistics. Health, United States, 2006, with Chartbook on Trends in the Health of Americans. Hyattsville, MD: 68–71.

Chapter 4

Page 77: Roughly 70 percent of veterans of OIF/OEF who report some kind of painful condition also say they have poor or unrefreshing sleep. Clark, M.E., Pain and Emotional Problems Among OIF/OEF Veterans. Slide show presentation.

Chapter 6

Page 125: In one study, 100 percent of those who used the therapy for four weeks had a significant decrease in their pain, as measured with two types of pain scales: Chan B.L., et al., Mirror Therapy for Phantom Limb Pain. NEJM 357:2206–2207, 2007.

Page 125: In one study of three amputees, overall phantom pain was cut in half, and the burning component of the pain was eliminated. Bittar A.G., et al., Deep Brain Stimulation for Phantom Pain. *J. Clinical Neuroscience* 12(4): 399–404, 2005.

Chapter 7

Page 139: A 2002 survey found that about 15.2 million adults in the Unite States alone have used yoga to help improve their health. National Center for Health Statistics and the National Center for Complementary and Alternative Medicine study of the use of complementary medicine techniques. National Institutes of Health, NCCAM Publication No. D412, 2008.

Chapter 8

Page 151: According to the U.S. Department of Veterans Affairs, about 6 to 11 percent of veterans of OEF, and between 12 and 20 percent of OIF veterans have been diagnosed with PTSD. United States Department of Veterans Affairs. National Center for Posttraumatic Stress Disorder Fact Sheet: How Common is PTSD? Available at www.ncptsd.va.gov/ncmain/ncdocs/fact_shts/fs_how_common_is_ptsd.html; accessed: 2/26/09.

Acknowledgments

I would like to thank the following people for their contributions, without which this book would not have come to fruition:

⊗ My wife Andrea, thank you for being there with support and guidance through the difficult and joyous times. You stood by and supported me during many questionable and uncertain moments. I am grateful for your service as a wife, mother, and veteran. Your journey and accomplishments are truly remarkable. I am blessed to have you as my wife, and I love you.

⊗ To my boys Sean and Ryan, thank you for saving my life! You gave me the motivation to live, recover to my fullest, and to be a father who will always support you. If you both take anything from this, know you can accomplish and overcome anything in your lives. Please know how much I love you both, and always will.

⊗ To my parents Dave and Barbara, thank you for the love and support you have given me throughout my life. I cannot imagine the many tireless nights of worry and concern you have had for my well-being. Without the quality of character you raised me to have I could not have overcome the difficulties and struggles in my life.

⊗ To Brenda Murdough, MSN, RN-C, for helping to create the concept, providing guidance and clinical expertise, and for her courage in standing up before Congress to testify in support of the Military and Veterans Pain Care Acts. Your understanding, passion, and commitment to caring for members of the military, veterans, and family members continue to provide inspiration and have made their mark in history.

❂ To Carolyn Noel, for your tireless efforts toward this project, your "eagle eye" in editing, your knowledge and guidance of both the military and website development, and your advocacy for other Marines, women, veterans, and fellow people with pain.

❂ To Tamara Sloan Anderson, MSW, for founding the Military and Veterans Pain Initiative at APF, for guiding the project and holding it together, for motivating and connecting people, for developing support for this work, and for working tirelessly on behalf of persons living with pain. Your dedicated passion for the military and veterans communities makes a difference in countless lives daily.

❂ To Rollin (Mac) Gallagher, MD, MPH, for your medical expertise, your commitment and care of veterans, and your guidance and constant support of the American Pain Foundation's efforts, and particularly the Military and Veterans Pain Initiative.

❂ Colonel Chester C. (Trip) Buckenmaier, III, MD, for your guidance and support, your passion about improving battlefield medicine and pain care, and for your service, both individually to this country and to the many service members who have been in your care.

❂ To the American Pain Foundation staff and volunteers—past, present and future—thank you for giving me a voice and a platform to share my story, and for helping to ensure that others don't have to suffer in silence from untreated or undertreated pain.

✪ To all the service members and veterans who have shared their stories and voices and joined us in our fight to improve pain care: without you, we wouldn't have passed the military and veterans pain legislation; and without you, we can't keep fighting to improve pain care. We're in this together.

✪ To all the dedicated healthcare providers who treated me as a whole person, listened to me, spent countless hours supporting me physically and emotionally while both on and off duty, who went above and beyond the call of duty: you helped me rebuild my life and, by extension, that of my family as well.

✪ To all those who use this book: it's worth the fight— keep going, keep fighting, don't give up, live life to the fullest, never surrender. I'm there with you.

The American Pain Foundation

The American Pain Foundation (APF) is the largest and most active pain patient organization in the country, serving the estimated 76.5 million Americans who suffer from pain. Since 1997, APF has worked alongside consumers, health-care professionals, regulators, families, and others to broaden the understanding of pain and increase access to quality pain treatment. APF's mission is to improve the quality of life of people living with pain, by raising public awareness, providing practical information, promoting research, and advocating to remove barriers and increase access to effective pain management. APF works in three main areas: Education and Support, Advocacy, and Research.

APF began the Military/Veterans Pain Initiative in 2004 in response to communications that we received from veterans suffering with pain from prior wars, and because of the growing number of veterans returning from Iraq and Afghanistan who were living with persistent pain. APF's initiative works to improve pain care on both a national level through legislation and policy, and an individual level, through education and support. In 2008, APF successfully led the fight to pass the Military and Veterans Pain Care Acts into law. These laws include critical provisions for pain care policy improvements from the battlefield to the Veterans Administration and beyond. Please join us in our efforts to improve pain care for members of the military and veterans.

The Exit Wounds Website

As an online companion to the *Exit Wounds* book, www.exitwoundsforveterans.org provides up-to-date information, education, and support for service members, veterans, and their families. The website follows the structure of book to give additional detailed information, and resources, as well as opportunities to interact with the author, fellow veterans, and pain management experts.

To Hell and Back

Scuttlebutt: Read, comment, and subscribe to this weekly blog from Derek McGinnis.

Amputee Information: Get updates on latest research and treatments.

Voices of Veterans: Hear other inspirational stories from veterans, and share your own.

Pain Management Tips: Find more tips on pain management, drawn from the American Pain Foundation's extensive Pain Information Library.

Coming Home in Pain

Resources: Access an up-to-date listing of available resources.

OEF/OIF Veterans: Learn about unique challenges faced by returning OEF/OIF veterans.

Chats & Webinars: Participate in live chats and webinars, or listen to the replay.

Online Support Group: Participate in APF's PainAid Online Support Community, where there's a special section reserved for military and veterans.

Exercise: A Key to Pain Relief

Sports & Recreation Resources: Refer to the listing of available civilian and military resources.

Upcoming Events: Review current events and share those happening in your area.

Getting Help

Invisible Injuries: Read about the relationship of PTSD, depression, and TBI to pain.

Financial Issues: Get information on navigating the DoD and VA medical systems, types of financial assistance available, and much more.

Family & Caregivers: Get information on navigating the DoD and VA medical systems, types of financial assistance available, and much more.